THE NEUTROPHIL

THE
NEUTROPHIL

Patrick Murphy

The Johns Hopkins University School of Medicine
Baltimore, Maryland

SPRINGER SCIENCE+BUSINESS MEDIA, LLC

Library of Congress Cataloging in Publication Data

Murphy, Patrick, 1937-
  The neutrophil.

  Includes bibliographical references and index.
  1. Neutrophils. I. Title. [DNLM: 1. Neutrophils. WH200 M978n]
QP95.8.M87   612'.11822   76-29077
ISBN 978-1-4684-7420-6   ISBN 978-1-4684-7418-3 (eBook)
DOI 10.1007/978-1-4684-7418-3

© **1976** Springer Science+Business Media New York
Originally published by Plenum Publishing Corporation in 1976
Softcover reprint of the hardcover 1st edition 1976

Dedicated to
Dr. I. Calma, Professor R. A. Gregory,
and Dr. T. G. Richards

Preface

This book reflects the personal prejudices I have developed in twenty years of reading the scientific literature. I like monographs; good ones assemble a great deal of information in a logical sequence and in enough detail to enable one to see why current beliefs are held. For this purpose, it is entirely useless to write "as Smith has shown[21,81,117]. . . ." That only means that one must go to the library and turn up Smith's original papers, and one's object in reading a monograph is precisely to avoid that necessity. One needs to know what Smith did and why he thought his observations proved whatever he claimed. Because life is short, it is impossible to deal with several thousand papers in this way, and the author must therefore select a relatively few papers that he regards as crucial. Often, several papers of equal merit might be quoted, and the selection is then arbitrary. I therefore apologize to authorities who do not find their work discussed. Omission does not mean that I thought their work was not valuable; it means only that I preferred to quote twenty references that people might read rather than two thousand that assuredly no one would read.

Another strong prejudice is that the full understanding of present knowledge requires one to know how present views have developed. Any reading in the old literature leaves one with a profound respect for the minds of the research workers of the time; only their technical resources were inferior to ours. Thus, I have had no hesitation in quoting Wright and Douglas (1903) as the reference for serum opsonins; anyone who bothers to go back and read the paper will at once see why. Elsewhere, I have in general preferred to quote the original observation rather than the very latest paper on the subject. However, I have indicated recent review articles and monographs when they were available; they serve as entry points to recent literature.

I included a section on inflammation because I found that my own graduate students did not have even a rudimentary knowledge of the process and presumed that other Ph.D. students in immunology were similarly ignorant. For the same reason, there are sections on kinins, the complement sequences, and chemotactic agents. Those who are acquainted with these matters can pass over those sections.

I would like to acknowledge a profound debt to Dr. Leon P. Weiss, who decided that I could write this book, suggested it to me, gave advice at all stages of writing, including two readings of the entire manuscript, and contributed many illustrations. However, I have not dedicated it to him; the single most important influence on my scientific character was Professor R. A. Gregory and the staff of the Department of Physiology at Liverpool University. They taught me to think, and whatever merits the book may have are primarily attributable to them. I did not even consider dedicating the book to my wife; she is an independent person with her own achievements, and she does not need reflected glory.

Several other people helped me to write this book. Dr. Hyun S. Shin read Chapter 5 and corrected some of my misunderstandings of his work. Dr. Manfred M. Mayer and Dr. Arthur M. Dannenberg, Jr., read several chapters, and both contributed helpful advice. I am also grateful to the investigators in other institutions who were so generous about contributing illustrations of their work. Several of them also sent me preprints and reprints of their latest results so that the book could be as up to date as possible; I especially wish to thank Drs. John Spitznagel and Marco Baggiolini. Lastly, I would like to thank my secretary, Ms. Lily E. Cowan, who heroically reduced my illegible manuscript to neatly typed pages, and patiently bore with me during numerous revisions.

P. M.

Baltimore

Contents

Chapter 8
Other Activities of Neutrophils **177**

Introduction

Modern immunology has so changed its emphasis that the neutrophil is rarely considered as anything other than an effector cell of no intrinsic interest. The chief concern of immunologists at present are the exploration of the ways in which antigen-responsive cells are stimulated by foreign materials, and of the consequences that flow from these interactions. There is no evidence to suggest that the neutrophil plays any part in the development of new capacities by immunized animals. Like the legendary jackass of Missouri, he is of uncertain ancestry and without hope of progeny, and there is no mechanism by which the experience of an individual neutrophil could be translated into altered function on the part of its descendants. Rather, the neutrophil is an end cell, with an impressive assortment of preformed antibacterial systems, that has a half-life in the blood of a few hours, and that survives in the tissues for at most a few days. It has virtually no capacity to adapt or improve its bactericidal mechanisms, and its improved performance in immune animals depends on antibodies that are manufactured by other cells. Nor does the neutrophil display much discrimination; given a suitable stimulus, it responds in the same stereotyped fashion whether the outcome be destruction of an invading parasite or of host tissue.

This unflattering picture of a disposable cell responding blindly to instructions is incomplete. There are very few bacteria that can evade the neutrophil when they are introduced into the tissues in anything less than overwhelming numbers. Indeed, for many organisms the lethal dose of living bacteria is of the same order of magnitude as the lethal dose of dead ones, and death is presumably due to toxins rather than to bacterial multiplication. The vital importance of the neutrophils is underlined by the fact that no man or animal can survive for longer than a few days without them. Experimentally, it is easy to show that animals deprived of neutrophils have greatly lessened resistance to almost any pathogenic bacterium. However, the infections that develop spontaneously in neutropenic animals are usually caused by bacteria that normally live on their skin and mucous membranes. Antibiotics are available which may prevent invasion by those members of the normal flora, such as staphylococci and gram-negative rods, that are occasional pathogens. In this case, death will result from infection with antibiotic-resistant organisms that are almost never pathogenic under normal circumstances.

Immunity originally meant the ability to resist infectious disease, and for this the neutrophil is vital. After all, the best media for growing bacteria are various soups and digests of animal tissues. It is true that the mononuclear phagocytes constitute a separate, and very important, system of phagocytic cells that are uniquely capable of dealing with certain organisms which defeat the neutrophil. In some regions of the body, mononuclear phagocytes constitute the front line; the first defense of the lung is the alveolar macrophage. The two types of cells complement one another, and both are essential for life.*

The idea that bacteria are disposed of by being taken up and digested by phagocytic cells is less than a century old, and was first clearly formulated by the Russian zoologist Elie Metchnikoff.[1] In his *Lectures on the Comparative Pathology of Inflammation,* delivered at the Pasteur Institute in 1891, he presented a summary of his early work, and his phagocytic theory of immunity was presented in full in his *Immunity in Infective Diseases,* of 1901.[2] It was based on an enormously broad knowledge of zoology that enabled him to make detailed comparisons between phenomena observed in the simplest of animals and those observed in man. He pointed out that phagocytosis in unicellular organisms was a feeding mechanism, although sometimes a bacterium ingested by a protozoon might multiply within its cytoplasm and a would-be meal developed into a lethal infectious disease. As multicellular organisms became more complex, there was a progressive tendency for digestion to occur extracellularly in a digestive tract. In most metazoa, only mesodermal cells retained the ability to phagocytose; they would congregate around a site of injury and take up

---

*That they are is not formally proved, because no man or animal congenitally deprived of macrophages has ever been described, and there is no convenient experimental method of producing one.

any microbes they found there. This cellular aggregation occurred in animals without a vascular system, but if there was a circulation, phagocytic cells were mobilized from the bloodstream. When bacteria were taken up by a phagocyte, they were usually killed and digested. Sometimes, however, they would survive intracellularly and might even multiply and destroy the phagocyte. Failure of phagocytes to eliminate bacteria at the site of invasion usually led to unrestrained multiplication of the microbes and death of the host. Metchnikoff therefore contended that phagocytosis was the main defense of multicellular organisms against disease.

This conclusion was hotly disputed by those responsible for the early triumphs of immunization against infectious disease, where immunity seemed clearly to depend on serum factors. In 1890, von Behring and Kitasato showed that the sera of immunized animals could neutralize tetanus toxin, and soon after they repeated the experiment with diphtheria toxin.[3] In 1894, Pfeiffer observed lysis of cholera vibrios by immune serum.[4] With the separation of antibody and complement activities by Bordet in 1895,[5] the way seemed clear for a totally humoral explanation of bacterial destruction.

Over the next ten years, the disputes were largely settled. Wright and Windsor showed in 1902 that human serum had little or no effect on several common pathogenic bacteria,[6] and this finding was rapidly confirmed by others. Leishman, in 1902,[7] described a method for quantitating the uptake of bacteria by human neutrophils, and in 1903, Wright and Douglas used it to show that human leukocytes would not phagocytose staphylococci unless normal plasma or serum was added to the mixture.[8] If the serum was heated at 60°C for 15 min, the power to promote phagocytosis was lost. The power was also lost if sera were allowed to age, or if they were treated with "viper venom." Finally, Wright and Douglas immunized a patient with sycosis barbae (an infection of the beard area) with his own staphylococci. The phagocytic power of the blood was much increased, and they showed that this effect was due to a change in the serum, not in the phagocytic cells themselves. They christened the new activity an *opsonin,* from the Greek "to prepare food for."

It was quite clear to Wright and Douglas' contemporaries that the heat-labile opsonin might be the "complement" that was known to participate in the lysis of erythrocytes and certain bacteria by immune sera. Muir and Martin, in 1905, demonstrated that complement fixation, or destruction of complement by any means, abolished the opsonic power of serum.[9] Since complement was known to require antibody for its action, it was logical to suppose that normal serum contained low levels of antibody to common bacteria. That it does was demonstrated in 1906 by Bulloch and Western, who showed that the opsonic power of normal sera for staphylococci could be absorbed out with the homologous organism, while leaving the opsonic activity for the unrelated *Pseudomonas pyocyanea* unchanged.[10] The cooperation of antibody and complement in the opsonic activity of normal sera for staphylococci was clearly nailed down by Cowie and Chapin, in 1907.[11]

The case of opsonic activity in the sera of specifically immunized animals appeared to be different. Neufeld and Rimpau, in 1904, showed that these sera opsonized in very high dilutions, and that heating at 56°C either did not affect the activity or reduced but did not abolish it.[12] This conclusion was soon confirmed by others. Thus, specific antibody appeared to be able to opsonize at least to some extent without the participation of complement.

It is amazing how little we have advanced since these experiments of seventy years ago. Metchnikoff was clearly right in his main proposition, although for a time he maintained that any opsonic factors in serum were produced by phagocytic cells. In modern terminology, the antibodies in normal sera are present in low titer, and are predominantly of the IgM class, which can opsonize only with the participation of complement. The antibodies in the sera of highly immunized animals are of the IgG class, and do not require complement for opsonization. Metchnikoff could only speculate on how phagocytic cells destroyed bacteria; we now know a large number of possible mechanisms, and we have some ideas about which are important *in vivo*. However, there are a host of factors that we can treat only in descriptive terms. We have no clear idea of where the enormous numbers of neutrophils that leave the circulation each day are deployed. We do not know what stimuli induce them to stick to vessel walls, or to insinuate themselves between epithelial cells. We can describe, as Metchnikoff did, the way in which they move in a quasi-purposive manner toward bacteria (chemotaxis), and we have some elementary knowledge of the chemical mediators that impel them to do so. But we do not understand the mechanisms of ameboid motion, still less the way in which it is rendered directional. We write confidently of "receptors" on the surface of phagocytic cells that recognize immunoglobulin and complement components, but we have no idea of their structure or indeed of their specificity. The precise way in which the phagocytic vacuole is formed has been elegantly displayed, but not the mechanisms by which the neck is closed and the membrane connection with the exterior severed. We do not understand why membrane fusion and degranulation occur, although we can observe the process, and its results.

Answers to this type of question require fundamental advances in cell physiology. Until they are obtained, we will continue to be confronted with occasional patients who are plagued with recurrent bacterial infections that we are unable to explain in any meaningful way. We can make phenomeno-logical observations of the kind that their neutrophils move slowly, or not at all; that they fail to respond to chemotactic stimuli; or that degranulation fails to occur—but there the matter ends. It is improbable that only work on neutrophils can provide the needed information; the whole thrust of modern biology emphasizes the fundamental unity of all living things, and it goes against the grain to suppose that a particular mammalian cell type has unique modes of operation. Certainly, it is not a hypothesis that would have appealed to Metchnikoff.

1

Blood Cells

About half the volume of normal blood is occupied by cells. By far the greater proportion of these cells are the *erythrocytes,* which contain hemoglobin and are responsible for the red color, and the principal function of which is oxygen transport. One or two per thousand cells in blood are colorless, and are known as *white cells,* or *leukocytes.* Stained blood smears show that there are six types of cells in blood besides the red cells. The appearances of these six types are illustrated in Figs. 1.1 and 1.2, and their relative proportions and absolute counts are given in Table 1.1.

1.1. Platelets

The most numerous cells are the *blood platelets,* which are not usually included in the term "leukocytes." They are small discoid objects measuring 2–3 μm in diameter and containing a few nondescript granules. Their principal function is in the prevention or stopping of bleeding.

1.2. White Cells

Nucleated *white cells* are divided into cells having a single nucleus that is not subdivided, and cells with segmented nuclei. The *mononuclear cells* also differ from the *polymorphonuclear cells* in that their cytoplasm does not contain obvious granules.

1.2.1. Lymphocytes

The most common mononuclear cells are the *lymphocytes.* They appear to be almost all nucleus in the light microscope, with just a thin rim

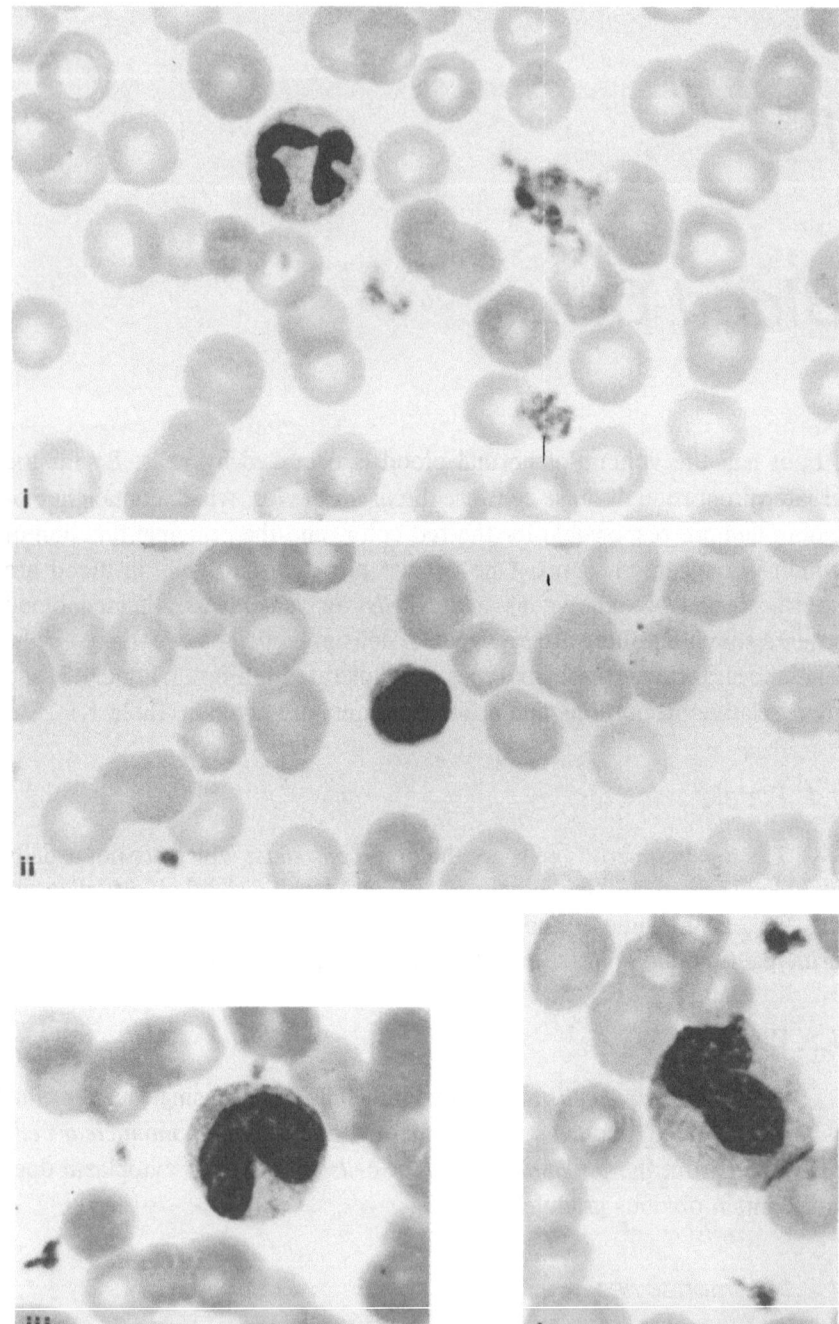

TABLE 1.1. Normal Proportions of Leukocytes in Peripheral
Blood Smears from Adult Humans

(Figures are cells/mm.³ Data adapted from *Hematology*, by Williams, Beutler, Erslev, and Rundles, McGraw–Hill, 1972. Used with permission of McGraw–Hill Book Co.)

Cell type	Mean number	Range of normal
Segmented neutrophils	4200	1800–7000
Band neutrophils	220	0[a]– 700
Eosinophils	200	0[a]– 450
Basophils	50	0[a]– 200
Lymphocytes	2500	1000–4800
Monocytes	300	0[a]– 800

[a]Because it is customary to count 100 cells, and at most 500 cells, when obtaining differential counts, cells that occur in small numbers may be missed due to sampling errors. However, it is not really normal to have no eosinophils, basophils, or other types of cells.

of pale blue cytoplasm. Despite their very uniform appearance, we now know that cells with this morphology may be committed to very different pathways of development. Some have matured in bone marrow *(B cells)*, and are destined to synthesize antibody. Others have matured in the thymus *(T cells)*, and will participate in cellular immune reactions of diverse types. Within these broad groups, subdivisions can be recognized. Thus, T cells comprise at least three separate populations of cells: those that are long lived and recirculate through the thoracic duct, those that are shorter-lived and tend to seek out inflamed areas, and "suppressor" T cells. The first group mediate immunological memory and allograft rejection, the second is concerned with defense against certain intracellular parasites such as the tubercle bacillus or *Toxoplasma gondii,* and the third is concerned with the regulation of immune responses. Furthermore, some cells that look like lymphocytes are not involved in immunological reactions, but are the precursor cells for granulocytes and other blood cells.

1.2.2. Monocytes

Monocytes are rather large mononuclear cells with a kidney-shaped nucleus and abundant cytoplasm. By light microscopy, the cytoplasm does not have much structure; there may be a foamy appearance. Supravital

←——————————————————————————————

FIG. 1.1. Blood films (Wright's stain, ×1400). (i) A single neutrophil with just discernible granules lies among erythrocytes and three small clumps of platelets. (ii) A small lymphocyte; the cell is almost all nucleus. (iii, iv) Monocytes. (Preparations supplied by Dr. C. Lockhard Conley.)

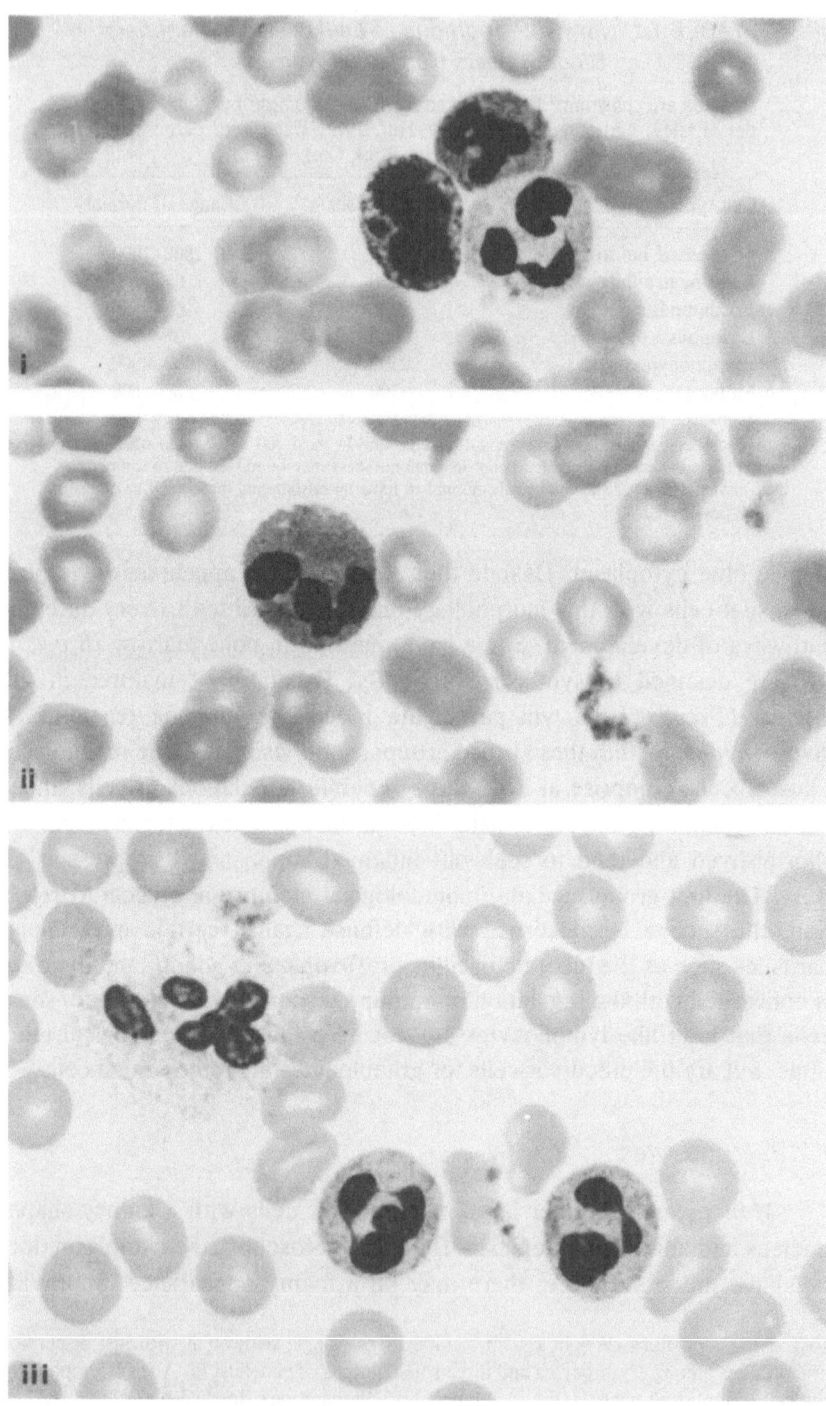

staining with certain dyes, such as neutral red, shows small vacuoles in monocyte cytoplasm. Monocytes are phagocytic cells that can take up and destroy microorganisms in their own right. In addition, they are the precursors of all the macrophages of the body, and when differentiated ("activated"), their powers of killing microorganisms are much increased. In some areas, macrophages are normally present and are renewed quite slowly; examples are the alveolar macrophages of the lung and the Kupffer cells of the liver. In other areas, there are only a few resident macrophages in the tissues, but monocytes rapidly enter from the blood once infection occurs, and in the tissue they differentiate into macrophages. In most inflammatory lesions, the overwhelming majority of the macrophages have been recently mobilized from blood rather than produced locally.

1.2.3. Polymorphonuclear Cells

Cells with segmented nuclei are known as *polymorphonuclear cells,* or *polymorphs* for short. They are further subdivided by the granules found in their cytoplasm; the cells are alternatively known as *granulocytes.* The names applied to the granules, and by extension to the cells, reflect their appearance in human blood smears stained with Romanovsky dyes such as Wright's stain. This stain is a mixture of methylene blue and eosin; the methylene blue has been oxidized under carefully controlled conditions so that it contains a number of purplish oxidation products. Methylene blue and its derivatives are positively charged at neutral pH; eosin is negatively charged under the same conditions. Cellular constituents with strong negative charges will therefore stain blue or blue-black; DNA is responsible for the dark blue appearance of nuclei, and ribosomes are responsible for the pale blue of lymphocyte cytoplasm.

(a) Basophils. One type of granulocyte has large granules that stain deep blue-black with Wright's stain; they are said to be *basophilic,* and the cell is referred to colloquially as a *basophil* (Fig. 1.3). Its full name would be *polymorphonuclear basophil granulocyte.* The granules are black because they contain heparin, which has many strongly ionized sulfate

FIG. 1.2. Blood films (Wright's stain, ×1400). (i) Two neutrophils and a basophil. Note the coarse dark basophil granules. (ii) An eosinophil, with coarse uniform granules, which are bright pink. (iii) Two neutrophils and a (multinucleated) megakaryocyte. The latter gives rise to platelets by budding them off from its cytoplasm. It is most characteristically found next to the vascular sinuses in bone marrow, and occasionally becomes dislodged into the blood. (Preparations supplied by Dr. C. Lockhard Conley.)

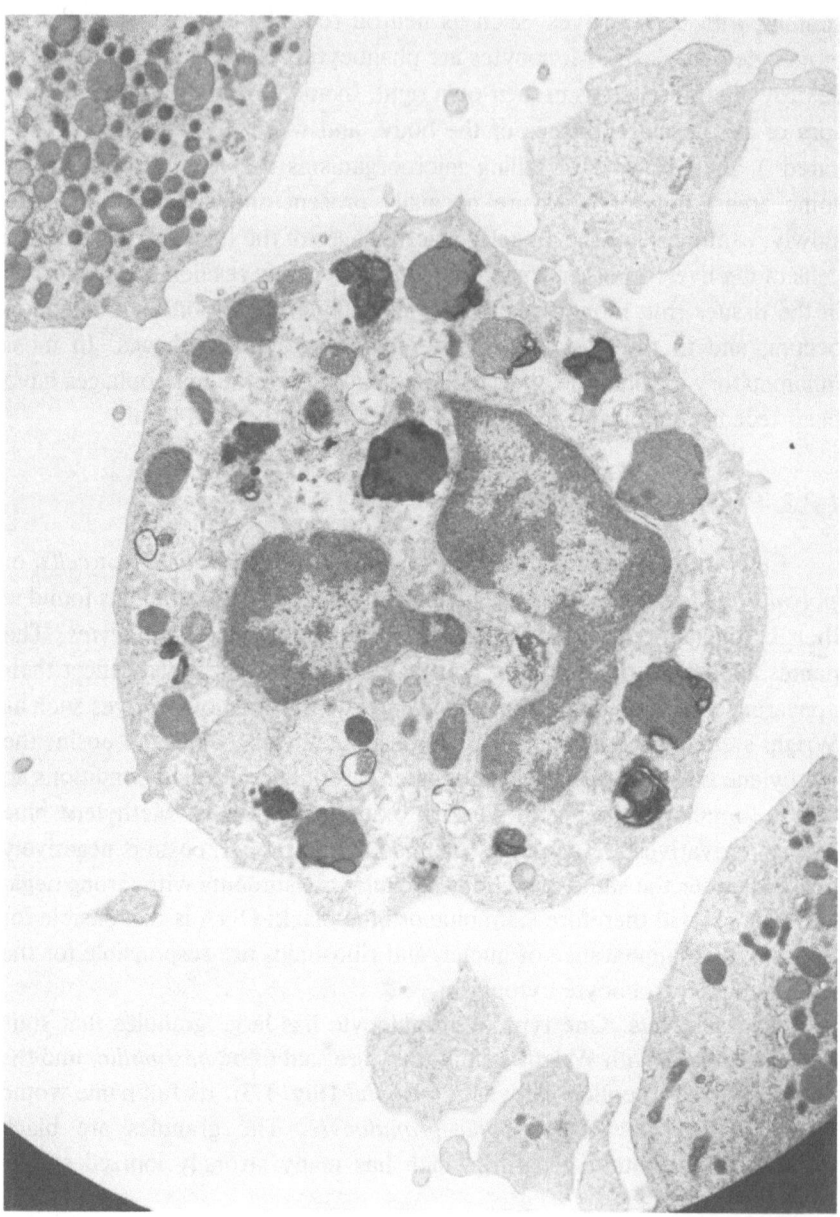

FIG. 1.3. Basophil from human blood, with portions of two neutrophils at top left and bottom right. Basophil granules are much larger and fewer than neutrophil granules, and are more varied in structure. Most show ordered crystalline arrays, but several also show folds of reduplicated membrane—"myelin figures." The Golgi region and the mitochondria are better retained than in neutrophils. [Picture contributed by Dr. Robin Hastie; see Hastie, R., A study of the ultrastructure of human basophil leukocytes, *Lab. Invest.* **31**:223 (1974).]

groups. They also contain histamine and other substances that cause contraction of smooth muscle and an increase in the permeability of small blood vessels. The function of the basophil is not known in detail, but it does participate in allergic reactions and is essential in some types of tissue damage such as serum sickness. Presumably, these pathological reactions are exaggerations of normal functions.

(b) Eosinophils. A second type of granulocyte has granules that stain red or orange with Wright's stain, and presumably contain some positively charged material. They are called *eosinophils* (Fig. 1.4). The function of the eosinophils is not known; however, they are dramatically increased in numbers during parasitic worm infestations. This increase is especially true when the worms are living in tissue, as in trichinosis; however, mild to moderate eosinophilia is characteristic of intestinal infections, such as hookworm, in which only the mouth parts are embedded in tissue.

Very recently, Warren and his colleagues have prepared antisera that were specifically directed against mature eosinophils. Mice treated with these sera had essentially no eosinophils in the peripheral blood, and were unable to accumulate eosinophils in the tissue lesions of schistosomiasis.[1] Such mice were also unable to develop the partial immunity to schistosomiasis that can be produced in normal animals.[2] The immunity appeared to have two components; the parasites were identified as foreign by antischistosomal antibody, and were then attacked by eosinophils. Mice treated with antisera against macrophages, lymphocytes, or neutrophils developed antischistosome immunity normally. If confirmed, these experiments are the first demonstration of a protective role for the eosinophil.

Eosinophils are also found under those epithelia that normally carry large bacterial populations, such as the nasal, intestinal, and vaginal mucosae. What they might be doing there is a mystery. They vanish from the blood during acute infections, but they may be found in inflammatory sites after a few days. They are not in the center of the lesion, but surround it at a respectful distance.

(c) Neutrophils. The most common granulocyte, the *neutrophil* (Fig. 1.5), is the subject of this monograph, and in man its granules stain neither red nor blue, but purplish. As we shall see, the granules of these cells contain many different substances; some carry strong negative charges, others carry equally strong positive charges. Furthermore, there are at least two different types of granules in these cells. Presumably, the overall balance between the different chemical constituents and the different granule types gives a net staining reaction that is about neutral. In some species,

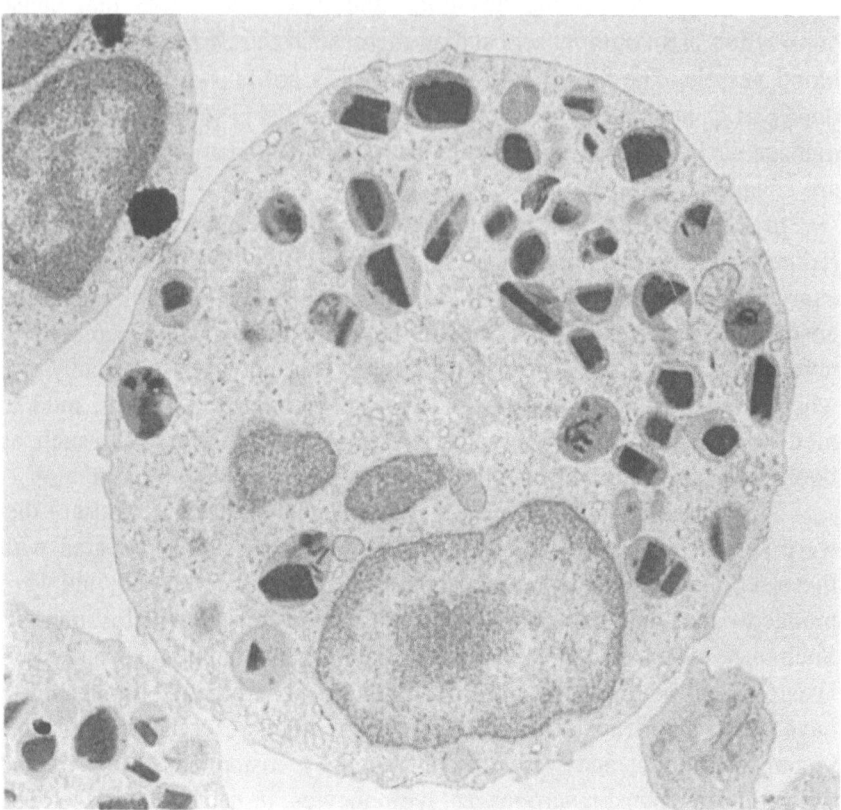

FIG. 1.4. Human eosinophil (electron micrograph). Note the large granules with crystalline inclusions. In the rat, these crystalline inclusions are very uniform, but in human material, their shape is variable; some are long thin rods, others are almost cuboidal. The nature of the crystalline material is unknown, but these inclusions are thought to constitute the Charcot–Leyden crystals that are often found in the sputum of asthmatics. (Picture contributed by Dr. Dorothea Zucker-Franklin.)

such as the rabbit, the overall effect is such that the granules are definitely pink. For this reason, some authors object to the term neutrophil as a general term applying to this cell in all species. However, none of the alternatives proposed seems attractive, and most people know what one means by the term "neutrophil," even if the cell in the species under consideration does not have strictly neutrophilic granules: One means the most common type of granulocyte, the principal function of which is to combat bacterial infection.

It might well be thought that the distinctions drawn above among granulocytes with different types of granules are spurious. After all, Wright's stain is a mixture of components, the composition of which is not known in detail and the staining reactions of which are not understood. However, there is much other evidence to support the idea that the differences are real. Basophil and eosinophil granules differ from each other and from neutrophil granules in size, shape, and number, as well as in color. The cells can be clearly differentiated in the living state by phase-contrast microscopy, and electron micrographs show that the internal structure of the granules is unique for each cell type (Figs. 1.3–1.5). Furthermore, it is unlikely that these cells represent different stages of development of the same cell line, or that they represent physiological

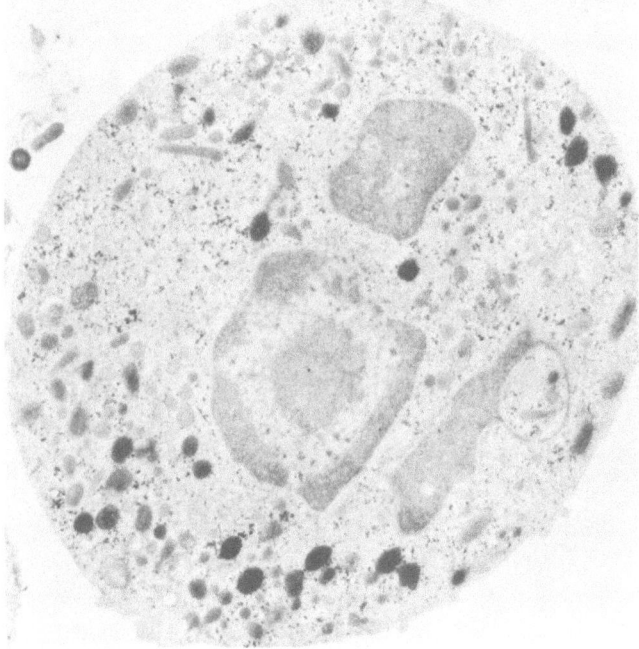

FIG. 1.5. Human neutrophil from blood (electron micrograph). The dark-staining granules are azurophils; they are usually shaped rather like a football. The light-colored granules are specific; they are mostly round, but some rodlike forms can be seen. The small black dots are glycogen granules. The Golgi region is inconspicuous, and mitochondria and endoplasmic reticulum are difficult to find. [From Bainton, Ullyot, and Farquhar, *J. Exp. Med.* **134:**907 (1971).]

variants of the same cell. The differences in granule staining and morphology can be recognized in bone marrow precursors back as far as the myelocyte stage, and there is no evidence of transitional forms.

Selected Reading

Wintrobe, M. M., *Clinical Hematology,* 7th ed., Lea & Feibiger, Philadelphia, 1975.
Williams, W. J., Beutler, E., Erslev, A. J., and Rundles, R. W., *Hematology,* McGraw–Hill Book Co., New York, 1972.

2

Morphology and Cellular Physiology of Neutrophil Granulocytes

Mature neutrophils, as found in normal blood, are very uniform cells with a diameter of 12–15 μm as measured in smears on glass slides. In tissue, the cells are rounded (presumably) and appear somewhat smaller. They are highly differentiated and have some unique structural features.

2.1. The Nucleus

The nucleus is subdivided into a number of lobes, usually two to five. It used to be thought that a cell with a multilobed nucleus was older than a cell with only two, but this idea is almost certainly false. Very young cells show a nucleus that is elongated and often twisted upon itself ("band" or "stab" cells). In normal blood, where cells are constantly leaving and new ones from bone marrow are replacing them, there is an equilibrium state with relatively constant proportions of young and old cells. During infections, tissue demand for neutrophils is high, many young cells are mobilized from bone marrow, the proportion of immature cells in the blood rises, and the differential count is said to show a "shift to the left" (Table 2.1).

The functional significance of nuclear segmentation is uncertain. Metchnikoff thought that it allowed the cells to emigrate from blood vessels more easily. However, both lymphocytes and monocytes seem to have no difficulty, and evidence for neutrophils suggests that cells with different

TABLE 2.1. Classification of Peripheral Blood Neutrophils by Number of Nuclear Segments and Maturity of Mononuclear Forms

(Proportions expressed as percentages. Modified from Wintrobe, *Clinical Hematology*, 7th ed., Lea & Feibiger, Philadelphia, 1975, by conflating the Arneth and the Schilling classifications.)

	Nonsegmented nuclei				Segmented nuclei (number of lobes)				
Condition	Myelo-blasts	Myelo-cytes	Metamyelo-cytes	Juveniles	2	3	4	5	>5
Normal	0	0	0.2	5	35	41	17	2	0
Infection[a]	0	0	0.5	30	60	9.5	0	0	0
Leukemoid reaction	0	2	10	50	30	8	0	0	0

[a]The response to infection is illustrative; the left shift may be smaller or larger. In general, severe infections are associated with higher neutrophil counts, greater degrees of left shift, and the presence of abnormal neutrophils with vacuoles, toxic granules, or Döhle bodies.

numbers of nuclear lobes leave the circulation at the same rate. Also, there is a congenital anomaly, the Pelger–Hüet anomaly, in which nuclear segmentation in neutrophils does not occur. Life expectancy is normal, and there is no obvious functional defect.

2.2. Nucleic Acid Metabolism

The nuclear chromatin is coarsely clumped, suggesting that much of the genome is inactive. There is virtually no incorporation of tritiated thymidine into cellular DNA, agreeing with the general view that these cells are end cells that do not divide.

There is no morphological evidence of a nucleolus in mature neutrophils. Biochemical evidence about RNA metabolism is rather unsatisfactory, because it is derived from blood cell populations that contain lymphocytes and monocytes, and one cannot be certain which cell type was responsible for the phenomena observed. However, populations that were mostly neutrophils (85%) did show incorporation of tritiated uridine into RNA. There were three pools: a 28 S + 18 S lightly labeled pool, presumably ribosomal; a 4 S rapidly labeled pool, presumably tRNA; and a rather heterogeneous, rapidly labeled pool thought to be mRNA.[1]

In interpreting these results, it would seem unlikely that neutrophils really can synthesize ribosomes, since they lack the organelle (the nucleolus) in which ribosomal synthesis occurs. However, there is evidence that neutrophils can synthesize certain proteins from amino acid precursors, and for this synthesis, the amino acids would have to be activated, and messenger RNA would be required. Actual synthesis of mRNA and tRNA is therefore plausible, though not absolutely proved.

2.3. The Cytoplasm

2.3.1. Carbohydrate Metabolism

Electron micrographs show that several types of granules and organelles are present in the cytoplasm (Fig. 1.5, p. 15). There are large numbers of small electron dense particles that are thought to be composed of glycogen. Neutrophils do contain large quantities of glycogen, as measured either by periodic acid Schiff staining or by extraction and chemical quantitation. It would seem that the major source of energy for the cell is glycolysis, an idea that is supported by the fact that the rate of glycogen breakdown is not greatly affected by oxygen; i.e., there is no Pasteur effect. Under normal conditions, the cell takes up glucose from its environment, and the glycogen content remains relatively constant. During phagocytosis, there are great increases in the rates of glycogen breakdown, glucose uptake, and lactate output, and total cell glycogen decreases.[2] We shall see later that phagocytosis cannot occur unless energy from glycolysis is available.

Mitochondria, and the enzymes of the Krebs cycle and electron transport chains, are present in mature neutrophils, but their numbers are relatively few (20–30 mitochondria/cell),[3] and it is uncertain how much of the cellular ATP is derived from this source. Certainly, neutrophils can move and take up bacteria in the total absence of oxygen. It is true that the bacteria may not be killed, but the reason appears to be failure of hydrogen peroxide generation under anaerobic conditions, rather than a shortage of high-energy compounds. Obviously, the ability to function effectively in the absence of oxygen is an advantage to a cell that must operate in inflammatory sites, where oxygen tension may be very low.

Neutrophils may also metabolize glucose by the hexose monophosphate shunt. Recent studies by Stjernholm and Manek show that only 1–2% of glucose metabolism proceeds by this route in the resting neutrophil, but that the quantity may rise to as much as 30% of total glucose utilization after the cell has phagocytosed bacteria (or small inert particles such as latex beads).[4] The first two steps of the shunt are dehydrogenation reactions that are obligately coupled to the reduction of NADP$^+$. Indeed, the cellular level of NADP$^+$ appears to control the overall rate of glucose metabolism by the pentose pathway. The NADPH is reoxidized by processes that are the subject of vigorous debate, and that will be discussed in detail in Chapter 7. However, it is clear that hydrogen peroxide is a major product, and that hydrogen peroxide generation during phagocytosis is crucial to several of the mechanisms by which neutrophils kill bacteria.

2.3.2. Protein Synthesis

The cytoplasm of neutrophils contains very little endoplasmic reticulum, smooth or rough. However, the mature neutrophil does retain some capacity for protein synthesis. Labeled amino acids are taken up and incorporated into protein, albeit at much lower rates than those seen in immature cells.[5] Polyribosomes can be isolated, presumably containing the messenger RNA, the synthesis of which was noted above.[6] As will be seen in Chapter 8, there is definite evidence that at least one protein is formed *de novo* from amino acid precursors when neutrophils are exposed to a suitable stimulus.

2.4. The Granules

The most prominent cytoplasmic constituents are the granules, which are visible by light microscopy and which have given the cell its alternative name of "granulocyte" (Fig. 1.5). There is considerable variation in granule morphology among species, but at least in the rabbit and in man there are two main types. The azurophil granules constitute 10–20% of the total population, and as the name suggests, they stain purplish with Romanovsky dyes. In electron micrographs of human neutrophils, they are dense, with a diameter of about 0.5 μm, and are surrounded by a unit membrane.

The specific granules are smaller (~ 0.2 μm), stain faintly pink, are relatively electron-lucent, and are also surrounded by a unit membrane. If the cells are homogenized in 0.34 M sucrose, a cloudy suspension of granules, nuclei, and other material results, and a relatively pure suspension of granules can be obtained by first sedimenting the nuclei and debris at low speed, then sedimenting the granules at high speed. Washed granules can then be placed on sucrose gradients, and centrifuged to equilibrium. Azurophil granules band at a density of 1.26, while specifics band at 1.23,

TABLE 2.2. *Enzymes in Neutrophil Granules*

[From Baggiolini, M., The enzymes of the granules of poly-morphonuclear leukocytes and their functions, *Enzyme* **13**:132 (1972).]

Enzyme	Species
DNAse II	Rabbit
Acid ribonuclease	Rabbit, horse, cattle
Lipase	Rabbit
Phospholipases A and B	Rabbit
Acid phosphatase	Rabbit, man, horse
α-Amylase	Man
α- and β-Glucosidases	Man
β-Glucuronidase	Rabbit, man, others
Elastase	Man
Neutral proteases	Rabbit, man
Collagenase	Man
Cathepsin D	Rabbit, man

with very little overlap between the two.[7] Thus, the enzymatic activities of the two types of granules can be examined separately.

Azurophil granules prove to be typical lysosomes, containing various hydrolytic enzymes with optimal activity at about pH 5. Some of the enzymes that have been found in azurophil granules are listed in Table 2.2, and it will be noted that collectively they are able to break down organic material into building blocks such as amino acids, sugars, and nucleotides. It is thought that these enzymes are responsible for disposing of the carcasses of dead bacteria; however, they are not in general lethal for living organisms. Enzymes that occur in azurophil granules and may actually kill bacteria are lysozyme and myeloperoxidase. Lysozyme hydrolyzes the muramic acid–*N*-acetyl glucosamine bond, which is found in the mucopep-tide coat of all bacteria (Fig. 2.1). Myeloperoxidase is an enzyme that is capable of complexing with hydrogen peroxide and using it to effect oxidations of various types. It may be present in huge amounts, up to 5% of the dry weight of the cell.

Azurophil granules also contain some nonenzymatic materials, two of which are of known biological significance. A group of proteins with highly positive charges, called *cationic proteins,* includes antibacterial substances and a protein that causes inflammation when injected into the skin. Also, there are sulfated mucopolysaccharides with highly negative charges. The

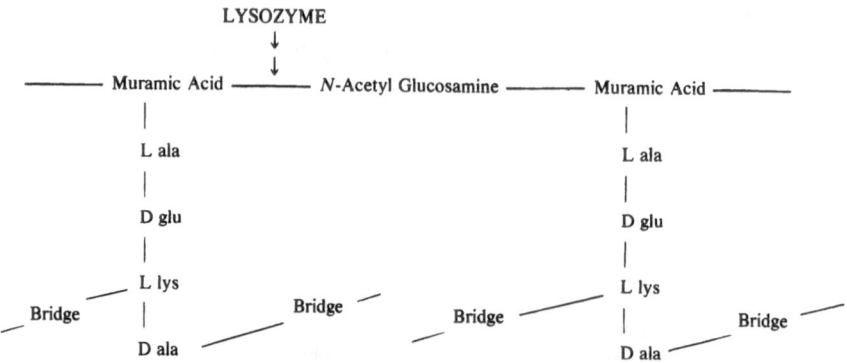

FIG. 2.1. All bacterial cell walls contain the backbone structure (muramic acid–N-acetyl glucosamine)$_n$. There is some variation in the amino acid side chain, but there is always a diamino acid at position 3 and a terminal D ala. The COOH group of the D ala residue is linked to the NH_2 group of the L lys residue by means of a bridge, which varies from one species to another. In *Staphylococcus aureus*, the bridge is (gly)$_5$; in *Streptococcus pyogenes*, it is (L ala)$_2$; in *Escherichia coli*, there is a direct COOH–NH_2 bond; and so on. This three-dimensional network gives strength and rigidity to the cell wall. Lysozyme disrupts the structure, and the unsupported cell membrane bursts under the internal osmotic pressure of the bacterium.

normal function of these substances is not known, but they are thought to have something to do with the generalized blood clotting seen in the Shwartzmann phenomenon (Chapter 8).

Specific granules also contain lysozyme and, in addition, lactoferrin. Lactoferrin is a protein that was originally found in milk and proved to contain a heme prosthetic group, hence the name. The protein in specific granules is immunologically identical with that in milk, and it has an extraordinary affinity for ferric iron.[8] All bacteria need iron to grow, and lactoferrin reduces free-iron concentration to far below the required levels. We shall see later that lactoferrin may also play a part in the killing of bacteria. It used to be thought that alkaline phosphatase was contained in specific granules, but two recent papers agree that this enzyme is associated with a microsomal fraction, and can be resolved away from lactoferrin.[9]

The ways in which neutrophils may utilize these various substances to kill bacteria will be discussed in detail in Chapter 7. The development of neutrophil granules will be taken up in the next chapter, but it may be said here that their contents are synthesized in the endoplasmic reticulum and packaged in the Golgi apparatus. This process occurs during the development of the cell in the bone marrow, and has ceased in the mature neutrophil. There is a Golgi region in the adult cell, but it is small, nondescript, and apparently inactive.

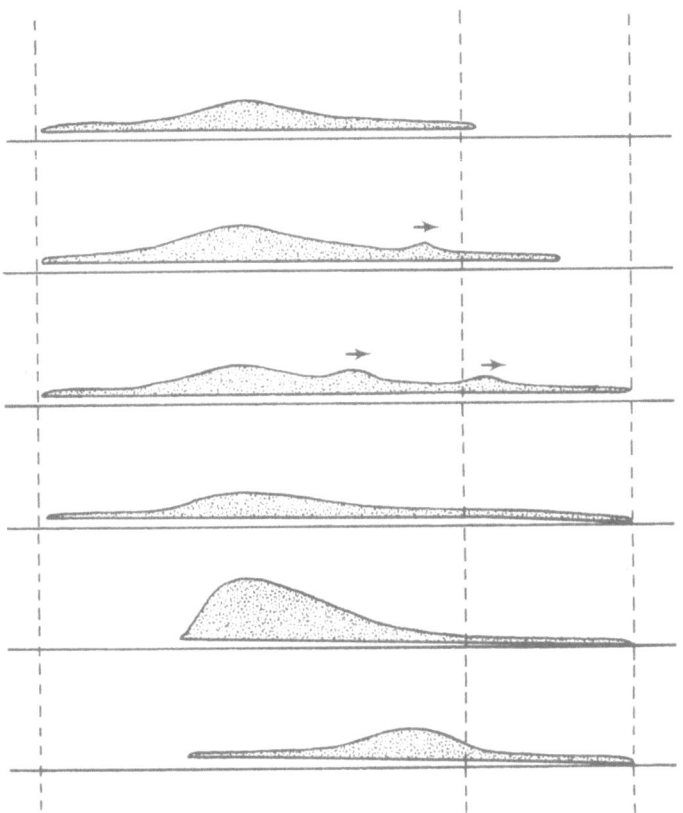

FIG. 2.2. The lamellipodial method of locomotion, as viewed from the side. [After Ramsey, W. S., *Exp. Cell Res.* **72**:489 (1972).[10]]

2.5. Cell Movement

The most characteristic activity of the living neutrophil is its mobility. This mobility is usually observed on glass slides; under these conditions, the cells put out a broad sheet of membrane, the *lamellipodium,* which is exceedingly thin but has the same width as does the entire cell. Initially, the lamellipodium contains no granules or other cytoplasmic constituents; these substances flow into it later. Cinemicrophotography of the process shows that the cells alternate between a completely flat, spread-out state, and a state in which the rear end detaches from the substratum and moves forward while the front end remains fixed.[10] In the latter stage, the cell becomes progressively rounded and protrudes into the medium (Fig. 2.2). Observation from the side shows that folds of membrane arise over the body of the cell, sweep down into the lamellipodium, and contribute to its extension. A cell may put out more than one lamellipodium; if it does, those directed away from the axis of cell movement do not fill with cytoplasmic granules. At the rear and side of the cell, the membrane appears to stick, and this sticking may leave behind long filamentous extensions *(retraction fibers),* which break as the cell continues to move away. This occurrence would imply that a constant supply of new membrane must be available to replace that lost by adhesion to the substratum.

This type of locomotion, in which the cell apparently takes a grip on the surface with its front end and then pulls the rear part forward, has been observed in fibroblasts. There are also some protozoa (Difflugia) that progress in this way. The motion does require a flat adhesive surface on which spreading can occur. Carter found that fibroblasts did not move at all on cellulose acetate membranes, but would do so if the membrane were shadowed with palladium. If the intensity of shadowing were varied gradually from one end of a membrane to the other, the cells crawled up the gradient toward the heavily shadowed end. They could also be induced to follow a narrow groove cut through the cellulose acetate film to expose the glass beneath.[11]

Recently, evidence from several laboratories has shown that neutrophils contain contractile proteins that presumably provide the motive force for their locomotion. It is thought that the morphological equivalent of the contractile proteins is the layer of microfilaments that lies underneath the cell membrane. It had been known for some time that if neutrophils were treated with glycerine to make the membrane permeable, they would contract in response to ATP. This behavior is also seen in skeletal muscle, and it suggested that neutrophils might contain proteins similar to actin and myosin. The first isolation of these proteins from neutrophils was reported in 1969 by Senda and his colleagues, who isolated the neutrophils from 9 liters of horse blood. The cells were homogenized in potassium chloride; the DNA was removed, and the actomyosin complexes were precipitated by adding ATP. The precipitate had ATPase activity, and examination in the analytical ultracentrifuge showed two peaks identical to those of skeletal muscle actin and myosin. Electron microscopy showed thick and thin filaments similar to those of skeletal muscle.[12]

Subsequently, Stossel and Pollard isolated myosin from guinea pig neutrophils and showed that it and skeletal muscle myosin ran as one band during SDS electrophoresis on acrylamide gel. The two proteins gave a reaction of identity when run against antiskeletal muscle myosin in Ouchterlony gels.[13]

Isolation of actin and myosin separately from the same neutrophils was achieved by Tatsumi and his colleagues using horse blood. Their actin formed helical filamentous structures with a pitch of 35 nm and a width of 7.5 nm, both values identical to those for skeletal muscle actin. It also coprecipitated with skeletal muscle actin in the presence of magnesium and ATP. The myosin appeared to resemble that of smooth muscle, rather than that of skeletal muscle, in that its ATPase activity was enhanced by calcium rather than magnesium and was more active at high ionic strength than low. The electron microscopic appearance showed filaments with a diameter of 15 nm, but a little shorter than those from skeletal muscle. Detailed analysis of the response of the actomyosin complexes to Ca^{2+}, Mg^{2+}, ionic strength, and ATP also suggested that the system resembled that of smooth muscle.[14]

Indirect evidence is provided by the actions of a fungal product, cytochalasin B, which has the property of disaggregating microfilaments and blocking the motility of ameboid cells. It does not block the motion of ciliates and flagellates, which depends on microtubules. Cytochalasin B at levels of 0.5–1 μg/ml blocks the motility of neutrophils and prevents the ruffling of the cell membrane.[15] Since it is known that actomyosin complexes provide the driving force for the motion of amoebas such as *A. proteus,* it would seem likely that the motility of neutrophils also depends on contractile proteins of the actin and myosin types. Unfortunately for this simple view, the actions of cytochalasin B on neutrophils are very complex, and low concentrations may actually stimulate motility. Also, it causes gross alterations in cell metabolism. Whether these other actions of cytochalasin B are primary or secondary remains to be worked out; in the meantime, the action of this drug in blocking motility can be regarded as only suggestive, rather than definitive. Cytochalasin B also prevents phagocytosis. Presumably, this prevention implies that the cytoplasmic flow around a particle is also mediated by contraction of microfilaments.

One may wonder whether the lamellipodial method of locomotion seen on glass slides is really representative of how the neutrophil moves *in vivo.* Glass is a very abnormal surface for a neutrophil, and the spread-out, pancake morphology of the cells probably reflects the strong adhesion between cell membrane and glass. It is difficult to believe that a method of locomotion by which the cell leaves a trail of membrane fragments behind it can possibly be physiological. It is also not easy to see how the cell could progress in tissue by means of an extension 8–10 μm broad. Certainly, neutrophils emigrate from blood vessels through openings less than 1 μm in diameter. Furthermore, their capacity to invaginate the periendothelial cells that surround capillaries would be much easier to explain if the motion were occurring as a consequence of hydraulic pressure generated by contraction of fibrils at the rear of the cell.

2.6. Directed Cell Movement

Chemotaxis is the capacity of a cell to move toward (positive) or away from (negative) a stimulus. In the case of neutrophils, the most attractive stimuli are bacteria. Chemotaxis will be discussed in some detail later; here I wish only to touch on what little is known of the mechanism. Neutrophils observed on glass slides in the absence of a stimulus move by a "random walk" mechanism; i.e., the cell moves in a given direction for a random interval, then changes direction and continues for a further random interval, and so on. For a large number of cells, the net movement from the origin is zero; for any individual cell, the distance it will move from the origin in a given time can be predicted statistically.[16] When neutrophils are observed in the presence of bacteria, neither the speed of movement nor the mean interval of time between changes of direction is altered. What seems to happen is that directions that would result in the cell moving away from the attractive stimulus are selected less often. Furthermore, Ramsey found that if the bacterial stimulus is transferred from the front of the leukocyte to the rear, the cell reverses direction almost immediately.[17] All this is quite unlike the mechanism for chemotaxis in bacteria, where changes in direction are suppressed in the presence of a rising concentration of an attractive substance, and where reversal of an established movement takes a little time.[18] It suggests that the cell may actually be capable of recognizing a concentration difference across its own length, although no plausible mechanism for doing this has been described.

Ramsey suggested that the function of the retraction fibers might be to provide the cell with a greater distance between receptors for chemotactic substances. He analyzed the response of neutrophils moving on glass in response to a gradient of cyclic AMP. The cAMP was contained in an agar cylinder at a concentration of 1×10^{-5} M. Since the diffusion constant for this simple molecule was known, it was possible to calculate how the concentration varied with time at various distances from the cylinder. If the cell was sensing a gradient across its own length, that was 16 μM, and the concentration difference across that length was only 0.026 $\times$ 10^{-6} g/ml at 10 sec. On the other hand, if the cell was sensing a difference across 43 μM, which was the distance from the front to the furthest point of the retraction fiber, the concentration difference was 0.055 $\times$ 10^{-6} g/ml, or more than twice as great. It was observed that the cells continued to move accurately toward the cylinder up to 30 min from the start of the experiment. At this time, it was possible to show that even the concentration difference from the front of the cell to the end of the retraction fibers had fallen to a point at which it was smaller than the random fluctuation in the concentration of molecules that could be predicted on thermodynamic grounds.[19]

Zigmond contributed a detailed analysis of the movement of neutrophils moving on glass toward a line of aggregated gamma globulin. She found that the ratio of the shortest possible path to the path actually followed varied from 0.61 to 0.97, with a mean of 0.85. Of all the cells, 65% never deviated more than 30° from the shortest path. She confirmed that the frequency of turns was not affected by the chemotactic agent; however, the magnitude of the turn was proportional to the deviation of the path from the shortest route, and the direction of the turn was almost always (15 out of 16 times) toward the gamma globulin line. In her experiments, it appeared that the cell could sense a gradient over its own length; 18 out of 20 cells putting out their *first* pseudopodium did so in the direction of the chemotactic stimulus. This finding excludes the retraction fiber hypothesis discussed above, and also disposes finally of the idea that the neutrophil might sum up its experience over time as do bacteria.[20]

2.7. Microtubules and Degranulation

Neutrophils also contain a skeleton of microtubules, which appear to direct the intracellular motion of the azurophil and specific granules after phagocytosis. We will see in Chapter 7 that the contents of these granules are delivered directly into the phagocytic vacuole by a mechanism that avoids their release into the neutrophil cytoplasm. This degranulation phenomenon is prevented by treating neutrophils with either colchicine or vinblastine, both of which prevent the polymerization of microtubule subunits into functional tubules. Degranulation is also prevented by agents that raise the intracellular levels of cyclic AMP. Neutrophils contain a protein kinase that can phosphorylate several proteins, probably including tubulin, and that depends for its action on cAMP.[21] It was hypothesized that cAMP may stimulate this enzyme to phosphorylate the tubulin subunits of micro-tubules, and prevent their aggregation.

Colchicine and vinblastine do not interfere with random movement of neutrophils. However, they do block the responses of neutrophils to chem-otactic agents, at concentrations as low as 0.01 or 0.1 μg/ml.[22] This finding suggests that while microtubules are not the primary moving force, they do play a part in allowing the cell to undertake asymmetrical movements. Certainly, cells treated with colchicine can be seen to ruffle all over the membrane, rather than in one place.

Allison has proposed a hypothetical scheme that enables one to inte-grate the various threads of knowledge about chemotaxis, phagocytosis, and degranulation.[23] He thinks that contact of the membrane with a bacter-ium or other particle may cause a local increase in sodium permeability that leads to depolarization. Apparently, there is some unpublished evidence that this depolarization may occur. Just as in muscle, the sodium influx leads to release of calcium from intracellular vesicles, activation of the ATPase activity of actomyosin complexes, and contraction of microfila-ments. In the case of a particle, the contraction leads to phagocytosis. Chemotactic agents cause the same response, but since there is nothing to phagocytose, directed movement results. Perhaps the local increase in permeability is mediated by Becker's serine esterase (discussed in Chapter 5).

This hypothesis is plausible, but there is one very old observation that if true would destroy it. In the old phagocytosis literature, it is generally accepted that phagocytosis proceeds just as well in isotonic KCl as in NaCl. In such a medium, the neutrophils would be completely depolarized, and there would be no sodium to carry an inward current.

Allison's second type of neutrophil response is an activation of mem-brane adenyl cyclase, a rise in intracellular cyclic AMP, increased protein kinase activity, and an interference with microtubular function that renders directed functions such as degranulation and chemotaxis impossible. Since the muscle system is not interfered with, phagocytosis and random motion are unimpaired.

It is clear that degranulation is not dependent on the muscle system, because it occurs in cells that have been paralyzed by cytochalasin B. In these cells, phagocytosis is blocked, and in consequence, the enzymes of the granules are discharged into the medium, where they may be measured quantitatively.

Weissman and his colleagues have used this system to examine the effect of cyclic nucleotides, and other stimuli that affect cyclic nucleotide levels, on neutrophil degranulation.[24] He found that a rise in intracellular cyclic AMP causes decreased degranulation. The neutrophil apparently possesses β-adrenergic receptors, which can be stimulated with epinephrine or isoproterenol and blocked by propranalol. Like β-adrenergic receptors in other tissues, they activate adenyl cyclase. α-Adrenergic agents had no effect on enzyme release. Neutrophils also appear to have receptors for histamine and for prostaglandin E_1; both these substances also raise the intracellular level of cAMP and caused reduced enzyme release. Cholinergic stimulation with carbamylcholine caused increased degranulation; this effect was blocked by atropine. Weissman found that cyclic GMP caused increased degranulation; whether the cholinergic effect was due to raised cGMP or to lowered cAMP was not determined. The involvement of the microtubular system in the process of degranulation was confirmed by showing that colchicine blocked it, and that deuterated water, which promotes microtubular formation, enhanced it. Weissman's results have been independently confirmed in Ignarro's laboratory.[25]

It is not absolutely clear that cAMP interferes with degranulation by preventing the aggregation of tubulin into microtubules. Weissman found that very low levels of cAMP (which are more likely to be physiological) actually stimulate phagocytosis and subsequent degranulation. He suggested that perhaps high levels of cAMP produce random aggregates of tubulin all over the cell, so that no "directed traffic" is possible.

2.8. The Cell Membrane

Last, we may discuss the cell membrane. In electron micrographs, it appears as a unit membrane similar to that of all other cells. Its appearance does not alter even though there may be considerable functional differences between the membranes of one neutrophil and another. Thus, cells that have phagocytosed organisms, or have been treated with bacterial endotoxin, become sticky and tend to clump together. They are also more efficient phagocytes, which may be another expression of the same phenomenon. Cells that have responded to a chemotactic stimulus are altered in that a serine esterase in their membranes is activated and then permanently deactivated. Many other such changes could be listed.

The cell membrane is consumed during phagocytosis because it is invaginated to provide a covering for the particle. The capacity of neutrophils for phagocytosis is uncertain, but cells containing 20–30 organisms are not hard to find in dense mixtures of bacteria and neutrophils. This amount of phagocytosis may well involve interiorization of half or more of the original surface area of the cell. It may also be that membrane is lost during cell locomotion, as was discussed earlier. There is biochemical evidence of fairly active membrane turnover in neutrophils, and of increased turnover and net membrane synthesis during phagocytosis. Simple compounds such as [^{14}C]acetate, [^{14}C]glucose, and [^{32}P]phosphate are incorporated into membrane lipids in the resting cell, and the rates are somewhat increased during phagocytosis. Detailed analysis of the lipids that become labeled reveals that most of the incorporation is into minor fractions (triglycerides and cholesterol), and that the phospholipids that compose 60–80% of membrane lipid are not labeled at all. This problem has been solved by Elsbach, who showed that the principal source for new membrane lipid is preformed lysolecithin, which is carried complexed to plasma albumin.[26] This lysolecithin is already phosphorylated—hence the absence of incorporation of ^{32}P—and it is converted to lecithin by addition of a preformed fatty acid molecule that is obtained either from plasma or by hydrolysis of cell triglyceride. Hence the absence of labeling with fatty acid precursors. Phosphatidyl ethanolamine and phosphatidyl serine are similarly synthesized from lyso precursors in plasma. Elsbach calculates that as much as 10% of the cell membrane may be renewed per hour, and that this rate is tripled during phagocytosis. If the cell membranes are prelabeled by incubating the cells with labeled lyso precursors before phagocytosis, it is possible to see whether membrane breakdown products accumulate in the medium at an increased rate. The answer is no, and it is therefore presumed that increased incorporation of lysolecithin during phagocytosis reflects net membrane synthesis.

That increased synthesis of membrane lipid from lyso precursors is important is suggested by the effects of the inhibitor levorphanol. This inhibitor is an analogue of morphine that was originally used by Gale to study membranes in bacteria. It can be shown to reversibly block the acylation of lysolecithin by intact neutrophils, though not, oddly enough, by disrupted cell fractions.[27] Cells treated with levorphanol show a reduction in phagocytic capacity ranging from 20% to 90%, depending on the particle tested, and degranulation is also blocked.[28]

Although there is clear evidence that neutrophils can to some extent replace the lipid components of lost membrane, it seems very unlikely that they can synthesize adequate quantities of the membrane proteins. The availability of these proteins is therefore the factor that will limit production of new membrane and ultimately phagocytic capacity.

It is possible to isolate phagocytic vesicles by feeding neutrophils a particle of low density, such as a latex bead. If the cells are carefully disrupted after phagocytosis, the vesicles can be separated out by differential centrifugation. It has been found that the lipids of phagocytic vesicles contain more saturated fatty acids (palmitic) and less unsaturated fatty acids (oleic and arachidonic) than are found in normal cell membranes. By prelabeling the neutrophils with ^{14}C-labeled fatty acids, it was possible to show preferential incorporation of saturated acids into phagocytic vesicle membranes.[29] Membranes with increased saturated fatty acid content are less permeable to water-soluble substances—an obvious advantage to a cell that pours highly destructive enzymes onto bacterial surfaces and would itself be destroyed if they were admitted to the cytoplasm. Elsbach has recently isolated phagocytic vesicles from neutrophils, and has shown, using radiolabeled precursors, that virtually all the lysolecithin taken up from serum by the cells is acylated and incorporated into the vesicle membranes.[30] This finding is direct evidence that the increased lipid synthesis is used to supply new membrane for wrapping bacteria.

It is currently thought that membrane proteins are not structurally bound in any particular arrangement, but float in the liquefied lipid bilayer and can redistribute themselves in response to various stimuli. Among the proteins found in neutrophil membranes are lectin-binding sites and proteins concerned with the inward transport of amino acids. Berlin has shown that binding sites for the plant lectin concanavallin A are preferentially incorporated into membrane areas that are being interiorized around a phagocytic particle. Conversely, amino acid transport proteins are preferentially excluded from vesicle membranes. After phagocytosis, neutrophils therefore bind much less concanavallin A than usual, but their capacity to transport amino acids is unimpaired. Both these redistributions are blocked by colchicine or vinblastine, although the number of particles interiorized remains the same. Presumably these redistributions of membrane proteins are other examples of an asymmetrical cell function mediated by microtubules.[31]

Selected Reading

Bessis, M., *Living Blood Cells and Their Ultrastructure,* translated by R. I. Weed, Springer-Verlag, Berlin, 1973.

3

The Origin and Development of Neutrophils

The information under this general heading is of three rather disconnected kinds. First, there is the classic morphological work, which traces the origin of blood neutrophils from myeloblasts in bone marrow, and physiological evidence about functional differences between mature and immature cells. Second, there is evidence about the kinetics of neutrophil production and utilization during normal and pathological states, which has been derived mostly from radioactively labeled populations of cells. Third, there are the attempts to find a more fundamental cellular origin for the neutrophil and other blood cells. We will take them up in this order.

3.1. The Bone Marrow and Neutrophil Precursors

Although the first blood cells are formed in the yolk sac of the embryo, and although at a subsequent stage of development the liver is a major site for hemopoiesis, the only important source for blood cells in adult animals is the bone marrow. Perhaps the best evidence that this is so comes from experiments with mice irradiated with doses of X rays sufficient to induce hemopoietic failure and rapid death due to infection. Such an animal will survive either if one of its legs is shielded from the radiation or if it is given a transfusion of normal bone marrow cells from a mouse with an identical genotype. The supporting evidence is vast and conclusive: Precursors of all types of blood cells can be seen in bone marrow preparations; their numbers and degree of activity correspond to spontaneous or induced

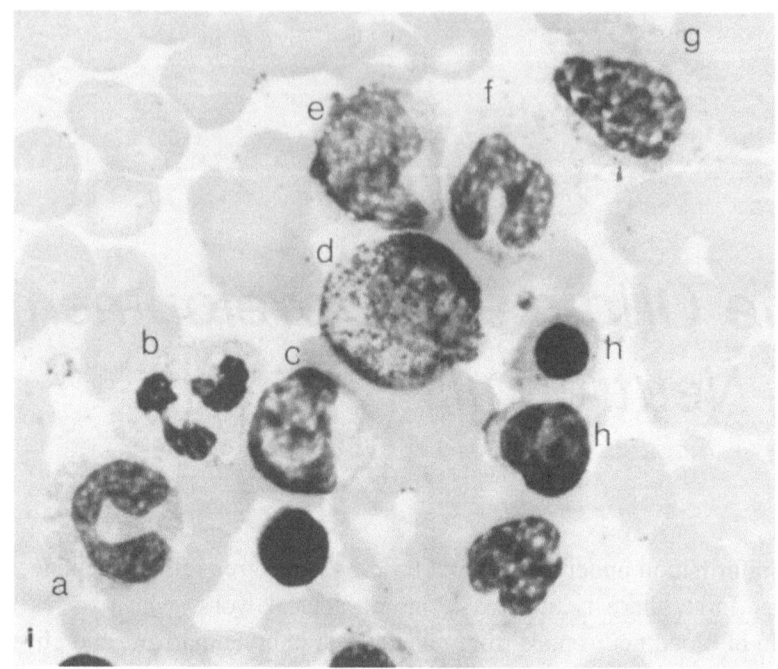

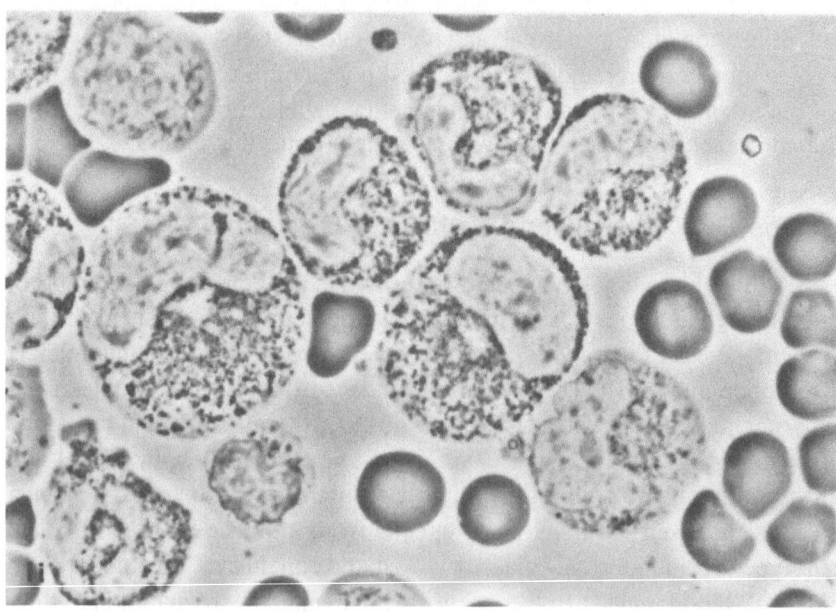

changes in the demand for particular cells; and diseases in which bone marrow is displaced by other tissue lead to a characteristic type of anemia in which nodules of hemopoietic tissue develop in unusual sites, such as the spleen.

Human bone marrow is usually studied by the examination of stained smears of material aspirated from some accessible bone with a thin cortex, such as the sternum or ileum (Fig. 3.1). In these preparations, a large number of apparently mature neutrophils can be seen, together with an at least equally large number of band cells. It is difficult to determine with precision the proportion of various cell types in bone marrow, because aspirated marrow is always contaminated with large amounts of blood and because it is difficult to secure adequately randomized samples of marrow particles. However, mature neutrophils and band forms together amount to about 25% of the total cell population, and it can be calculated that the bone marrow of an adult man contains about 30 times as many neutrophils as are present in the circulating blood. This marrow reserve can be mobilized very rapidly in response either to an infection or to the experimental injection of substances such as bacterial endotoxin.

The immediate precursor of the mature forms is a cell called the *metamyelocyte*. Here, as elsewhere, there is an arbitrary element in the categories to which cells in a continuous developmental sequence are assigned. Metamyelocytes shade into myelocytes at one extreme and band forms at the other. A typical neutrophil metamyelocyte is unmistakable, because the cytoplasm contains a full complement of granules. It can be clearly distinguished from basophilic and eosinophilic metamyelocytes in the light microscope, and in electron micrographs, the difference in granule morphology is particularly obvious (see Figs. 1.3–1.5). The cell nucleus shows extensive clumping of chromatin, and is indented or horseshoe-shaped. The metamyelocyte does not divide, and is not normally found in peripheral blood.

Preceding the metamyelocyte is the myelocyte. The myelocyte stage begins with the formation of the first specific granules, and ends when the

---

←

FIG. 3.1. (i) Human bone marrow smear (Wright's stain): (a) eosinophil metamyelocyte, (b) mature neutrophil, (c) myeloblast, (d) early myelocyte (note two sorts of granules), (e) late myelocyte, (f) neutrophil metamyelocyte, (g) myelocyte, (h) cells of the erythrocytic series. (Preparation courtesy of Dr. C. Lockhard Conley.) (ii) Human bone marrow, living cells (under phase contrast). Almost all the cells are neutrophil myelocytes and metamyelocytes. (Photograph contributed by Dr. G. Adolph Ackerman.)

cell has a full complement. Late myelocytes can be firmly classified as neutrophilic, eosinophilic, or basophilic because of the characteristic granules; classification is more difficult in earlier stages. All myelocytes can be readily distinguished from precursors of monocytes, lymphocytes, plasma cells, and so forth. The myelocyte is a fairly large cell, 16–25 μm in diameter, with a nucleus that is rounded and may be eccentric. The chromatin is mostly loose, though some clumping appears late in this stage, and one or two nucleoli are usually present. Myelocytes do divide, and 1–2% of cells in typical smears are in mitosis. Early myelocytes have deeply basophilic cytoplasm, but this is lost during the stage, and late myelocytes have faintly pink cytoplasm. Electron micrographs of late myelocytes show a few glycogen granules.

The earliest cell that can be identified with certainty as a neutrophil precursor is the *promyelocyte*. These are cells of rather variable size (15–20 μm) with a large, rounded, central nucleus, usually one or two nucleoli, and scanty, deeply basophilic cytoplasm. The diagnostic feature is the presence of azurophil granules, which can be recognized histochemically because of their characteristic enzyme content. In addition to the azurophil granules, the cytoplasm contains numerous mitochondria, a moderate amount of endoplasmic reticulum, and numerous single ribosomes.

Earlier still is the *myeloblast,* which is a rather small cell with a large nucleus, several nucleoli, and finely dispersed chromatin. The cytoplasm is scanty and basophilic, and contains mitochondria and endoplasmic reticulum, but no granules. It is not possible to distinguish with certainty between myeloblasts, which can differentiate into granulocytes, and monoblasts and lymphoblasts, the corresponding precursors of monocytes and lymphocytes. In marrow sections in which the normal cellular architecture has not been disturbed, blast cells may be presumptively assigned to one of the three categories by examination of their more differentiated surrounding daughter cells. On this basis, it has been suggested that lymphoblasts can be distinguished by the possession of a single nucleolus, and by a perinuclear clear area. However, in view of the accumulating evidence that all blast cells originate from a common stem cell, hair-splitting is unproductive.

There is no direct information about the metabolism of neutrophil precursors except for that derived from leukemic cells, which probably does not apply to normal cells. The following interpretation is therefore speculative. From the appearance of the myeloblast, one would suppose that it is an aerobic cell that derives much of its energy from oxidative

TABLE 3.1. Percentages of Neutrophil
Precursors in Normal Adult Bone Marrow

(Modified from Wintrobe, *Clinical Hematology*, 7th
ed., Lea & Feibiger, Philadelphia, 1975)

Cell type	Mean	Range
Myeloblast	2	0.3– 5
Promyelocytes	5	1 – 8
Myelocytes	12	5 –19
Metamyelocytes	22	13 –32
Mature PMN's	20	7 –30
"Lymphocytes"	10	3 –17

phosphorylation in its numerous mitochondria. Cytoplasmic basophilia is due to the ribosomes and endoplasmic reticulum necessary for protein synthesis. During the promyelocyte stage, the enzymes of the azurophil granules are synthesized; during the myelocyte stage, the enzymes of specific granules. By the end of the myelocyte stage, the cell is fully equipped with granules, and will not need much more protein synthesis during its brief life. Inactivation of the genome (clumping of chromatin) has begun; most of the mitochondria have been lost, and the cell is beginning to derive its energy from glycolysis; the ribosomes and endoplasmic reticulum have been lost, and the Golgi apparatus is less prominent. During the metamyelocyte stage, nuclear differentiation continues until the segmented form with heavily clumped chromatin is established, and the cytoplasm fills with the glycogen granules characteristic of mature forms.

Overall, granulocyte precursors constitute about 50% of all the cells in bone marrow. The proportions usually given for the various forms are: myeloblasts, 2%; promyelocytes, 5%; myelocytes, 12%; metamyelocytes and band forms, 22%; mature polymorphs, 20%. These figures, from Wintrobe's classic textbook, are in fact averages with a very considerable variance (Table 3.1). However, they suggested that a myeloblast gives rise to two promyelocytes, four myelocytes, and eight metamyelocytes, which then mature without further division. This simple view is almost certainly incorrect; it assumes that there is a simple linear sequence of development and that there is no possibility that a myelocyte, for example, might not mature, but might divide several times, giving rise to more myelocytes. It also assumes that the time spent in each stage is the same, and ignores the possibility that some cells may die. Unfortunately, it is easier to deride the hypothesis than to propose a simple and accurate alternative.

A possible solution of this problem using purely morphological methods is provided by the studies of Sin and Sainte-Marie.[1] The rat thymus contains islands of granulopoietic tissue, which appear to arise from very small numbers (one to eight) of myeloblasts. A single island contains cells of approximately the same degree of maturity—all promyelocytes, all myelocytes, and so on. Islands of primitive neutrophil precursors contain fewer cells than those composed of mature forms. Since the islands are entirely surrounded by thymic tissue, all the precursor cells in a single island can be classified and counted by the use of serial sections. If one assumes that no cells earlier than the mature neutrophil leave the islets, and that cell death is infrequent (it was not often seen), then the relative numbers of cells at each stage give estimates of the number of mitoses in the preceding stage. The experimental data were best fitted by a scheme of one cell division at the myeloblast stage, two at the promyelocyte, three at the myelocyte, and one at the metamyelocyte (in rodents, it would seem that the earliest metamyelocytes can divide once). Of course, there is no guarantee that hemopoiesis in the thymic environment is identical with that in bone marrow, but the overall picture is in reasonable agreement with estimates from radioautography discussed below.

3.1.1. Granule Formation

The process of cytoplasmic granule formation has been beautifully illustrated by the studies of Bainton and her colleagues.[2] These studies were conducted initially in the rabbit, and subsequently with human bone marrow cells. Normal human bone marrow was obtained from the ribs of patients undergoing thoracic surgery, and the granulocyte precursors were separated, concentrated, and fixed in glutaraldehyde. The fixed cells were incubated with 3-3'-diamino benzidine and hydrogen peroxide; wherever peroxidase was present, an electron dense reaction product accumulated. After this treatment, the cells were stained with uranyl acetate, dehydrated, embedded, and sectioned for electron-microscopic examination in the usual way. In promyelocytes, peroxidase staining was found throughout the endoplasmic reticulum, and in the perinuclear cisterna, the Golgi apparatus, and all the granules (Fig. 3.2). Peroxidase staining was concentrated on the inner, concave face of the Golgi apparatus, and it appeared that, as in the rabbit, the new azurophil granules were budding from this face of the Golgi. This sequence is similar to that seen in pancreatic cells, where potentially lethal enzymes are synthesized in the endoplasmic reticulum

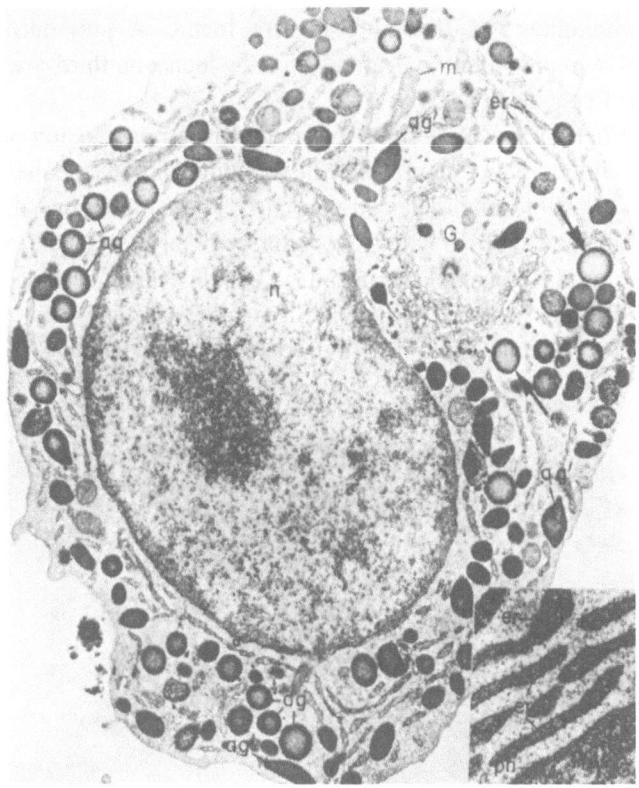

FIG. 3.2. A promyelocyte, reacted for peroxidase. All the granules stain darkly and correspond to the azurophil granules of mature forms. Many granules are spherical (ag); others are football-shaped (ag¹). Some granules have lighter centers (arrows), which may be an artifact due to inadequate penetration of the dye. The Golgi appartus (G), endoplasmic reticulum (er), and perinuclear cisterna (pn) are also stained, but no reaction product is seen in the nucleus (n) or mitochondria (m). [From Bainton *et al.*, *J. Exp. Med.* **134**:907 (1971).[2]]

and transported to the Golgi region, and move into the cytoplasm as membrane bound packets.

In the myelocyte, peroxidase staining had disappeared from all cell components except mature azurophil granules (Fig. 3.3). Granule formation was still active, but the granules were peroxidase-negative, and were budded from the outer, convex face of the Golgi apparatus (Fig. 3.4). Sometimes, myelocytes were seen which had a full complement of azurophil granules, but which showed no evidence of specific granule formation. In these cells, and perhaps in all cells, there was a complete halt between the formation of the two types of granules. Because azurophil granule formation ceases at a stage when the cell continues to divide, they are reduced in numbers in the more mature forms. A polymorphonuclear neutrophil contains about 200 granules, of which one-third are azurophil and the rest specific (Fig. 3.5).

The other enzymatic activities of peroxidase-positive and peroxidase-negative granules were determined histochemically, using methods that allowed both light- and electron-microscopic examination. Typical lysosomal enzymes such as acid phosphatase, or aryl sulfatase, were confined to peroxidase-positive (azurophil) granules, and were seen in promyelocytes. The peroxidase-negative (specific) granules that appeared at the myelocyte stage did not contain lysosomal enzymes.

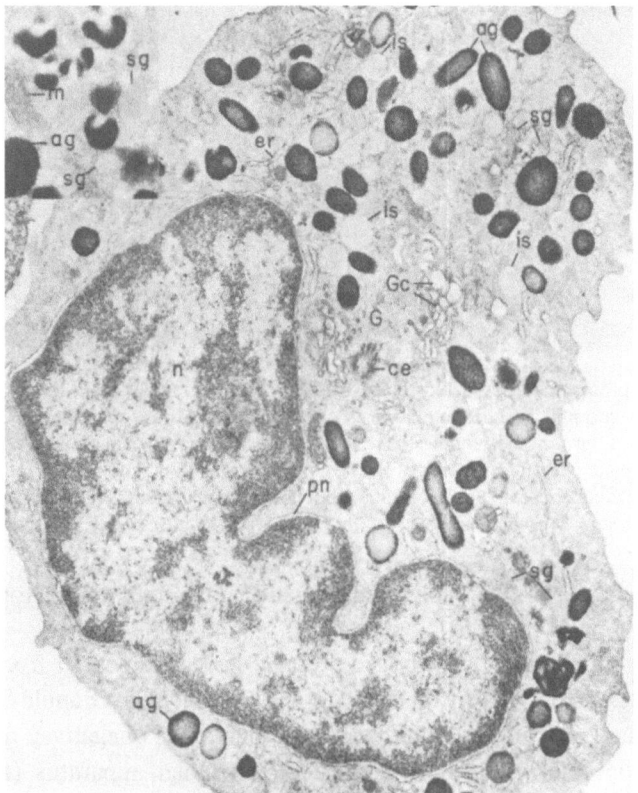

FIG. 3.3. A myelocyte, reacted for peroxidase. There are now peroxidase-negative specific granules (sg), as well as peroxidase-positive azurophil granules (ag). Immature specific granules (is), which are larger and more electron-lucent than mature specific granules, are found near the Golgi region (G). The endoplasmic reticulum (er), Golgi cisternae (Gc), and perinuclear space (pn) are free from peroxidase. (From Bainton *et al.*[2])

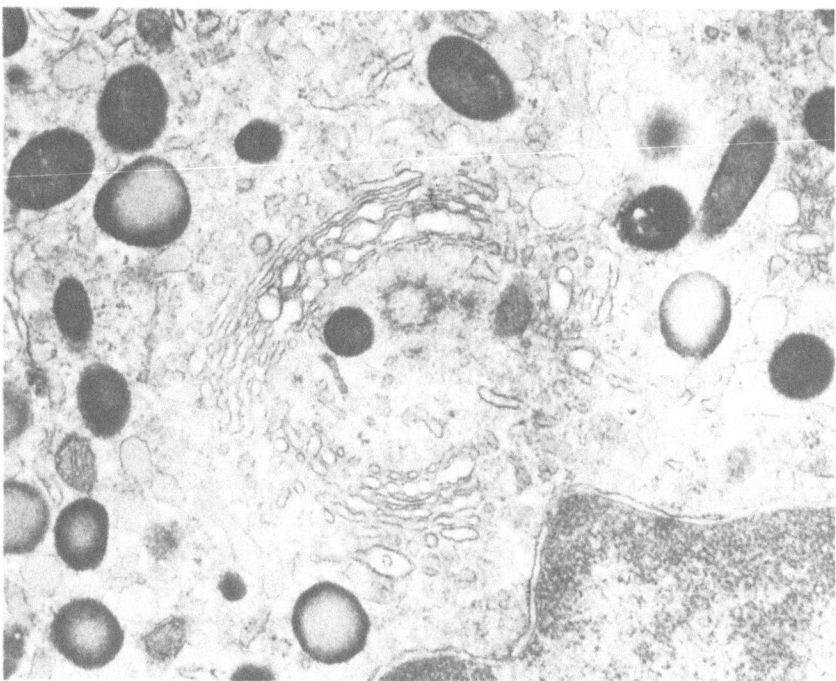

FIG. 3.4. Golgi region of a myelocyte (high-power view). The absence of peroxidase from the Golgi region, perinuclear space, and endoplasmic reticulum is confirmed. Tiny vesicles are budding from the outer surface of the Golgi cisternae; analysis of many such pictures suggests that they mature into specific granules. (From Bainton et al.[2])

3.1.2. Functional Differences Between Neutrophils and Their Precursors

It has long been known that there are great functional differences between neutrophils and their precursors. Immature cells move more slowly, respond poorly or not at all to chemotactic stimuli, and are relatively ineffective at phagocytosing microorganisms. Lichtman and Weed have recently made quantitative measurements of several of these properties and have correlated them with the degree of maturity as assessed morphologically.[3] Depending on the experiment, it was possible to classify cells into precise categories (myeloblasts, promyelocytes, and so forth), or into immature (myeloblasts through large myelocytes) and mature (cells with segmented nuclei). The adhesiveness of cells to glass was measured by suspending them in plasma, passing them through a small glass bead column, and comparing the proportions of various cell types in the effluent with the proportions put on the column. Another measure of adhesiveness

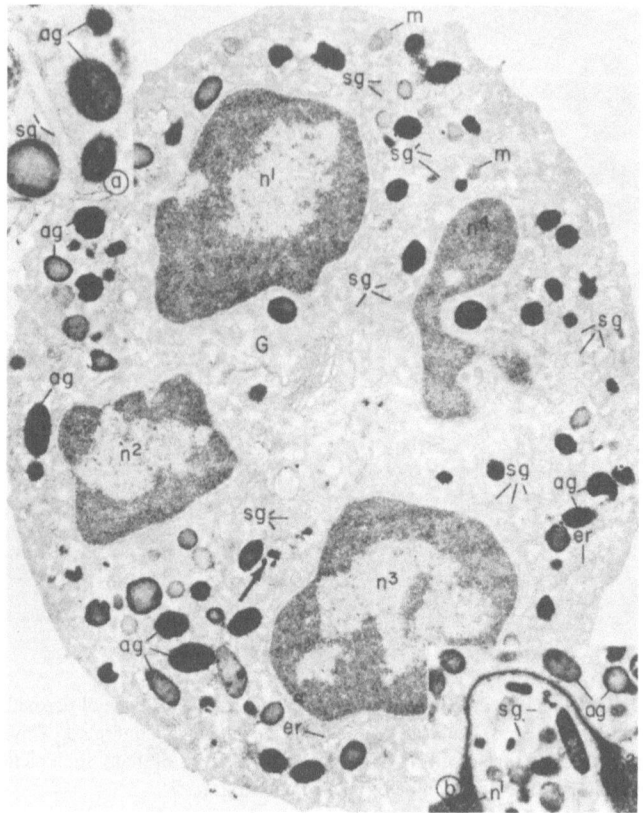

FIG. 3.5. A mature neutrophil, reacted for peroxidase. Most of the granules are specific (sg), because the azurophil granules tend to become diluted out. The nucleus has four lobes (n 1–4); one of the connections between the lobes is shown in insert (b). The Golgi region (G) is small and inactive, and the endoplasmic reticulum (er) and mitochondria are now difficult to find. Insert (a) shows some variants in granule size and shape; this variation explains why separation of granules by differential centrifugation is very difficult. (From Bainton *et al.*[2])

to glass was to allow cells to sediment onto coverslips for 15 min, then attempt to detach them by applying a 75–200g centrifugal force. Of mature neutrophils, 85% would resist such a force. The tendency of cells to stick to each other was measured by the progressive decrease in light-scattering when cells were incubated in buffered saline at 37°C. Mature cells clumped, precursors did not. Immature cells showed a somewhat higher electrophoretic mobility (a measure of net surface charge). The deformability of cells was assessed by measuring the negative pressure required to make a hemispherical knuckle of cytoplasm enter a micropipette with an orifice of

3.5 μm. This test showed a particularly clear differentiation in that once a mature neutrophil had been persuaded to put a hemisphere into the micropipette, it frequently followed with a pseudopod and eventually its whole self. This behavior was never seen with myeloblasts and promyeloctyes. Cell motility was studied by centrifuging them into a button in a capillary tube and measuring the rate of advance of the cell front. Mature neutrophils had an initial velocity of 400 μm/hr; immature forms, 60 μm/hr. Last, phagocytic ability was measured by suspending cells in plasma at 37°C, adding latex particles (diameter ~ 1 μm), and counting the number of cells that had ingested particles at various intervals. Myeloblasts and promyelocytes were virtually nonphagocytic, myelocytes intermediate, and all forms more mature than bands were efficient phagocytes. This last finding confirms a great body of evidence from other workers showing that there are no functionally significant differences between mature neutrophils with different numbers of nuclear lobes.

The differences observed could not be ascribed to the higher surface charge of the immature cell, because treatment with neuraminidase greatly lowered the surface charge without affecting any property except the electrophoretic mobility (neuraminidase is an enzyme that splits off negatively charged sialic acid from the glycoproteins and glycolipids of cell surfaces). It is not possible at present to make even a reasonable guess at the molecular basis for these striking differences in the cell periphery, but they are of obvious functional significance. To leave the bone marrow, a cell must squeeze through openings in the sinus wall with a maximum diameter of the order of 1 μm. These dimensions are similar to those of the holes in capillary walls by which cells leave the bloodstream for the tissues, and it is well known that in chronic myeloid leukemia, in which large numbers of immature neutrophils are found in the blood, the neutrophils that accumulate at sites of inflammation are almost all mature cells. Presumably, therefore, neutrophil precursors normally stay in the marrow because they are too rigid to get out. It is of interest that Weiss has recently shown that bacterial endotoxin, which leads to a mobilization of large numbers of neutrophils from the bone marrow, produces quite large apertures in the walls of marrow sinuses.[4] There is a large number of clinical conditions, both infective and noninfective, in which the neutrophil count is greatly elevated, and metamyelocytes, myelocytes, and even myeloblasts may appear in the bloodstream ("leukemoid reactions"). Whether these conditions have the same underlying mechanism is unknown.

The bone marrow vascular sinuses are lined by flattened endothelial

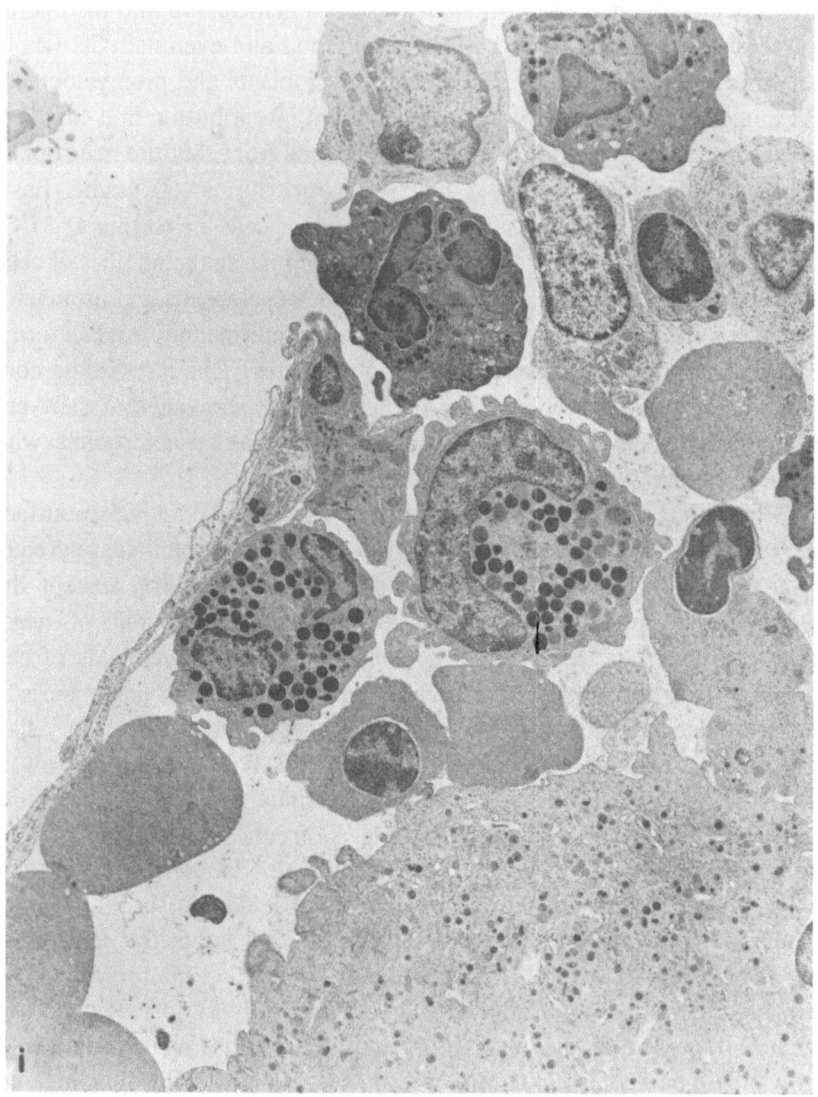

FIG. 3.6. Rat bone marrow (transmission electron micrographs of thin sections: (i) (×3650) Portions of two neutrophils are seen exiting from the marrow through the same aperture in the sinus wall. Two other neutrophils wait their turn just below them. The nonnucleated, homogeneous cells are erythrocytes; one late normoblast (erythrocyte precursor) is extruding its

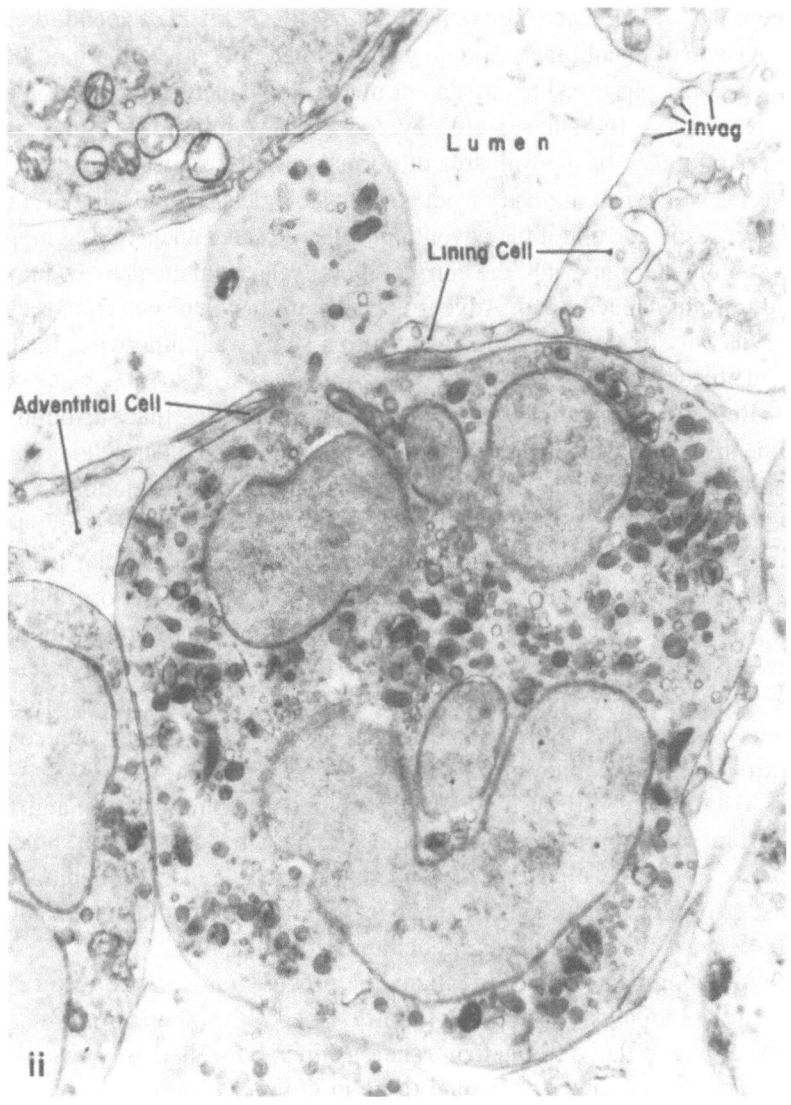

nucleus, while a second still retains it. The huge cell at the bottom right is part of a megakaryocyte. At the left, the sinus wall can be seen to be made up of a double layer of endothelium and adventitial cell; the basement membrane is not well seen in this picture. (ii) (×12,000) The earliest stage of neutrophil exit from marrow. (Pictures contributed by Dr. Leon Weiss.)

cells that are apposed by tight junctions. There are no gaps in the lining, except where blood cells are actually in passage. Outside the endothelium is a basement membrane containing a few small fibers, which are probably a species of collagen. This basement membrane is defective, existing only in areas where the sinuses are covered by adventitial cells. These cells cover about 60% of the wall area of normal vascular sinuses; the degree of covering can apparently vary from one physiological state to another, and it is easy to imagine that if the adventitial cells retracted and exposed more of the endothelial sinus wall, the entry of blood cells from the marrow into the blood would be facilitated. Adventitial cells are distinguished from recticular cells only by their position apposed to a sinus wall; otherwise, the cells are identical.

Reticular cells send out long branching processes that surround and define spaces in which the hemopoietic cells rest. Reticular cells probably secrete the extracellular fibrils that also surround the hemopoietic cells. The spongework of reticular cell processes is so pervasive that few if any hemopoietic cells are not contacted by it; indeed, the reticular cell processes may actually indent the cytoplasm of blood cell precursors, although there is no true cell-to-cell fusion. The intimate morphological relationship between blood cell precursors and the meshwork of reticular cell processes has suggested that reticular cells may not only provide an anatomical framework in which differentiation can occur, but also may induce and control that differentiation.

Macrophages are also widely distributed in bone marrow, and they send branching processes among the hemopoietic cells. Their function appears to be the phagocytosis and digestion of imperfect hemopoietic cells, or of unwanted organelles such as the nuclei of erythrocytes and the mitochondria and endoplasmic reticulum of neutrophils.

Although bone marrow contains the precursors of all the blood cells, they are not jumbled together haphazardly. Cells of similar ancestry tend to occur in groups that differ in their relationship to bone marrow sinuses (Fig. 3.6). Erythrocyte precursors tend to lie in groups close to the sinuses; as the cells mature into erythrocytes, the pyknotic nuclei and other organelles are extruded, while the erythrocyte passes through the sinus wall as a nonnucleated cell. Megakaryocytes characteristically lie directly apposed to the sinus wall; platelets bud off from cytoplasmic fingers that project into the lumen. Lymphocytes and monocytes are found in groups around the arteries. Neutrophil precursors occur in aggregates rather far removed from both the sinus wall and the arteries; only the later, motile, forms approach the sinuses and pass into the lumen. It seems likely that mitochondria and endoplasmic reticulum are extruded from the young granulocytes during this journey; they also develop microvilli—small fingerlike projections from the cell surface—which are well seen in Fig. 3.7.

3.2. Rates of Cell Division in Neutrophil Precursors

3.2.1. Morphological Methods

(a) Mitotic Time Method. Examination of the bone marrow by simple morphological methods can give useful information about cell turnover times. From smears, the numbers of myeloblasts, myelocytes, and other precursors can be determined; for each class of cell, the proportion in mitosis at any one time, the mitotic index, can be determined. It is assumed that normal bone marrow is a steady-state system, so that examination at any one time gives information that applies to all time. If the time each cell spends in mitosis, the mitotic time, can be determined, then kinetic data about neutrophil precursors can be obtained.

In animals, the mitotic time can be determined by the use of colchicine, which prevents the assembly of microtubules from their tubulin subunits. The mitotic spindle is not formed, and mitosis comes to a halt in metaphase. When bone marrow is examined at intervals after the drug has been given, mitotic figures increase steadily in number. Let us define the proportion of cells in mitosis at time 0, before the drug is given, as the mitotic index MI_0, and the index at some time, T, after the drug is given as MI_T. Let the time spent in mitosis be the mitotic time, T_m, and the total time between successive mitoses the generation time, T_G.

Now, clearly

$$\text{MI}_0 = \frac{T_m}{T_G} \quad \therefore T_G = \frac{T_m}{\text{MI}_0}$$

Let n be the total number of cells in the preparation. In the presence of colchicine, in any period of 1 hr, $(1/T_G)n$ mitoses will accumulate; and in T hr, $(T/T_G)n$ mitoses. The increase in mitotic index will be

$$\frac{T}{T_G} \cdot n \cdot \frac{1}{n} \quad \text{or} \quad \frac{T}{T_G}$$

So

$$MI_T = MI_0 + \frac{T}{T_G}$$

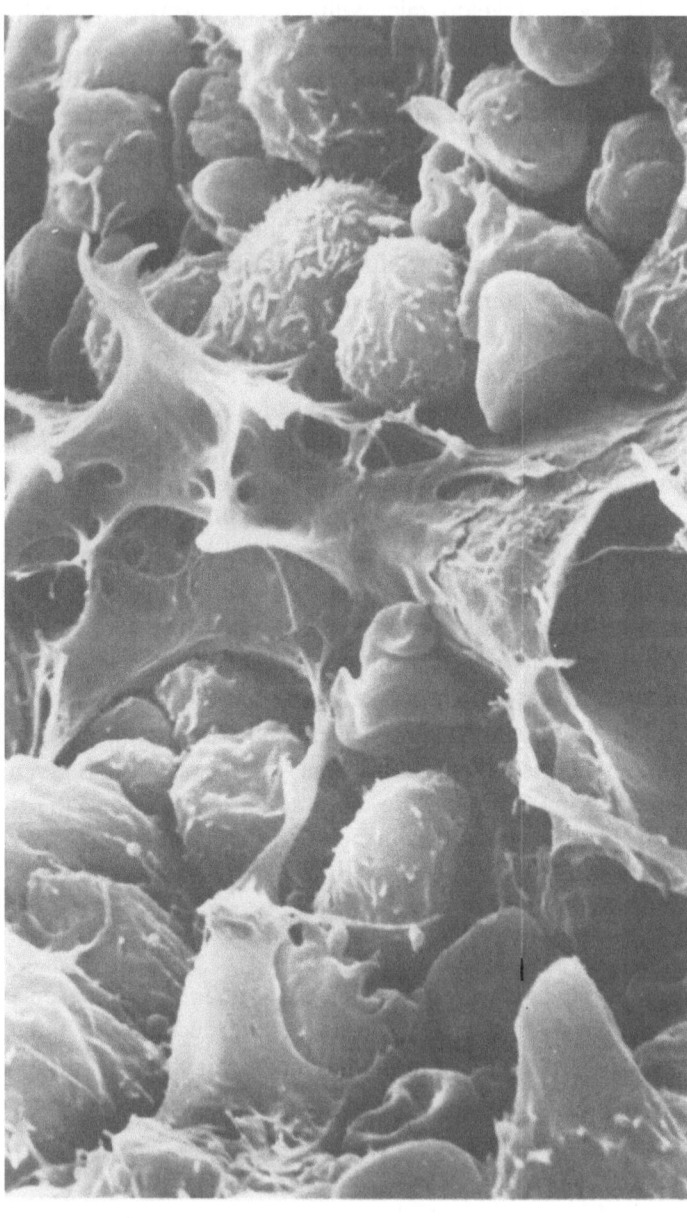

FIG. 3.7. Rat bone marrow (scanning electron micrograph). The lumen of the sinus is at the center bottom. The partial covering of the sinus endothelium by adventitial cells is well shown, as is the network of branching processes that surround and support the hemopoietic cells. The cells bearing microvilli are probably neutrophil granulocytes; the smooth, smaller ones are red cell precursors. (Photograph contributed by Dr. Leon Weiss.)

Substituting for T_G and rearranging,

$$T_m = \frac{MI_0 \cdot T}{MI_T - MI_0}$$

or if MI_0 is much smaller than MI_T,

$$T_m = \frac{MI_0 \cdot T}{MI_T}$$

and once T_m is known,

$$T_G = \frac{T_m}{MI_0}$$

Average figures are about 1 hr for mitotic time, and between 1 and 3 days for generation time, with the lower figures for myeloblasts and the higher ones for myelocytes.

Cronkite pointed out a fatal flaw in these calculations.[5] The assumption that $MI_0 = T_m/T_G$ is true only under two circumstances: (a) that each stage has only one mitosis, and that the daughter cells are immediately recognizable as some other type of cell; and (b) that no substantial number of cells in the compartment arises through maturation from an earlier stage, without cell division. With regard to (a), consider a hypothetical generation scheme in which a myelocyte divides into daughter myelocytes, which after a time, T_G, mature into metamyelocytes without further division. The original cell is visible in the marrow for a time, T_G, and the daughter cells, since there are two of them, for $2T_G$. There is only one mitosis in this time, occupying time T_m. The mitotic index is thus $T_m/3T_G$. With regard to (b), consider Cronkite's own example of the metamyelocyte compartment, where there is no mitosis, MI_0 is zero, and the generation time is infinite. There is a substantial turnover, which is entirely explained by the acquisition of cells from myelocytes at one end of the compartment and the loss of neutrophils to the blood at the other. The mitotic index method has other problems relating to cells that may be resting and not in active cycle, and the possibility that some cells may die without maturing.

(b) Compartment Transit Time Method. Cronkite's solution was to define a new parameter, the compartment transit time (C.T.T.), which is the average time from the entrance of a cell into a compartment until it or its progeny leave the compartment. In normal bone marrow, there is a steady-state situation in which the number of cells in, say, the myelocyte compartment remains static. The number of cells leaving the compartment must be

composed of two parts; one is clearly the number entering. If no mitosis occurs in the compartment, then $n_{in} = n_{out}$. Each mitosis adds one extra cell to the compartment (one of the daughters merely replaces the parent). Therefore

$$n_{out} = n_{in} + m$$

where m is the number of mitoses. This argument may now be carried forward. In compartment 1

$$n_{out(1)} = n_{in(1)} + m_1$$

But for compartment 2,

$$n_{out(1)} = n_{in(2)}$$

So

$$n_{out(2)} = n_{in(2)} + m_2$$
$$= n_{in(1)} + m_1 + m_2$$

And in general

$$n_{in(i)} = n_{in(1)} + m_1 + m_2 \cdots + m_{i-1}$$

Since the equations remain valid when divided throughout by any time t, the n's can be replaced by K's, which are the number of cells entering and leaving per unit time. There must be a stem cell compartment for which K_{in} is zero, so that

$$K_{in(i)} = m_1 + m_2 + \cdots + m_{(i-1)}$$

and if i refers to a compartment where there is no mitosis,

$$K_{in(i)} = K_{out(i)} = m_1 + m_2 + \cdots + m_{(i-1)}$$

In short, each mature neutrophil released to the blood is several generations removed from the stem cell compartment. However, the total number of such cells released over any long period of time is precisely equal to the number of mitoses that have occurred at all precursor stages combined during the same period of time.

An average value for the mitotic time was obtained from the observation that if tritiated thymidine was given, labeled metamyelocytes were found in the bone marrow within 3 hr, but not until 84 hr later were labeled neutrophils found in the blood. (Thymidine is a DNA label discussed in more detail below.) This 84 hr is presumably the metamyelocyte C.T.T. Of

1000 bone marrow cells, 361.4 were nondividing neutrophils, so that the number entering the blood in 1 hr must be 361/84 = 4.3. As discussed above, this must be the average mitotic rate for all precursor stages combined. At any one time, 2.5 per thousand bone marrow cells are in mitosis, so the mitotic time must be 2.5/4.3 = 0.58 hr. Let us assume that this average mitotic time applies to all precursors alike.

In the myeloblast compartment, we suppose that there is no cell entry; i.e., under normal circumstances, the myeloblast is the self-regenerating stem cell compartment. This supposition is probably untrue, but the flux of cells into the myeloblast compartment is thought to be small compared to the mitotic birth rate. Then, $K_{out} = K_m$, and the C.T.T. for a population N, is N/K_m. The mitotic index for myeloblasts is 24.9/1000 cells, and if the mitotic time is 0.58 hr, then the number of mitoses per 1000 cells per hr = 24.9/0.58 = 43, and the C.T.T. = 1000/43 = 23 hr.

From marrow differential counts, for each myeloblast there are 3.37 promyelocytes, so the size of the promyelocyte compartment corresponding to 1000 myeloblasts is 3370. The promyelocyte mitotic index is 14.8 mitoses/1000 cells, so that among 3370 cells, there would be 3.37 × 14.8 = 50 mitoses at any one time, and 50/0.58 = 86.2 mitoses/hr. One cannot calculate a precise C.T.T. for a compartment in which mitoses occur. However, the absolute minimum would occur when a cell entered the promyelocyte compartment, divided, and was immediately recognizable as a myelocyte. This minimum is given by $N/K_{out} = N/(K_{in} + K_m) = 3370/(43 + 86) = 26$ hr. The maximum would occur if there were no mitosis at all in the compartment, and would be $N/K_{in} = 3370/43 = 78$ hr.

By similar methods, transit time could be calculated for the myelocyte compartment; the maximum was 126 hr, and the minimum 37.4 hr. Cronkite's estimates would thus suggest a minimum overall time from myeloblast to mature neutrophil of 7 days and a maximum of 13 days.

3.2.2. Tritiated Thymidine Methods

More information can be obtained by the use of labeled thymidine. The immediate precursors of nucleic acids are the trinucleotides, which in the case of thymine would be thymine deoxyribotyl triphosphate. However, the three phosphate groups give the nucleotides a strong negative charge, and they penetrate cell membranes very poorly. The nucleosides do penetrate easily, and, once inside the cell, are phosphorylated and incorporated into RNA and DNA. Thymidine is a specific DNA label because RNA contains no thymine. Provided the level of radioactivity is not too high, no cellular damage seems to be produced by the internal radiation, and since DNA turns over very slowly, the cell and its descendants remain labeled until successive cell divisions have reduced the activity to background levels.

Dividing cells show a cycle of four more or less well defined phases (Fig. 3.8). M is mitosis, and following this is a period, gap 1 or $G1$, during which no DNA synthesis occurs. In the S phase, the genome is duplicated, and during this period, labeled thymidine will be taken up by the cell and incorporated into DNA. This uptake is usually detected by radioautography. After the S phase, there is a second gap, $G2$, during which the cell prepares for mitosis. After mitosis, a cell may enter the so-called G_0 phase, in which no preparations for DNA synthesis are made, and the cell is temporarily or permanently out of cycle. Obviously, the distinction between G_0 and a prolonged $G1$ is a matter of terminology, particularly since we have little idea what the cell does during $G1$.

(a) Grain Count Halving Method. The simplest technique depends on administering ^{3}H-labeled thymidine and observing the rates of disappearance of label from marrow cells and the appearance of label in the blood. There is good evidence that a single dose of thymidine is available for only 10–30 min after injection, so that only those cells in the S phase at the time of injection will be labeled ("flash" or "pulse" labeling). Each time a cell divides, the number of grains seen over the nucleus in radioautographs will be halved. This grain count halving time gives an upper limit for the generation time, the principal errors being due to the entry of heavily labeled cells from a previous compartment and to the presence of G_0, or nondividing cells. Both errors will produce a high estimated generation time.

Cronkite's estimates of grain count halving time in human bone marrow are: myeloblast compartment, 24 hr; promyelocytes, 24 hr; myelocytes, 54 hr.[6] In the myelocyte compartment, the grain count halving time was clearly inflated by the entry of labeled cells from the promyelocyte compartment, and probably by the presence of G_0 cells. Another estimate of generation time could be made by considering the partition of label between the large (early) and small (late) myelocytes. The large myelocytes had a high labeling index (L.I.) of 0.55–0.7, but small ones were less active, with an L.I. of 0.1–0.2. Labeled small myelocytes accumulated at 3–5%/hr, giving an estimate for T_G of 33–20 hr, and incidentally supporting the view that large myelocytes precede small.

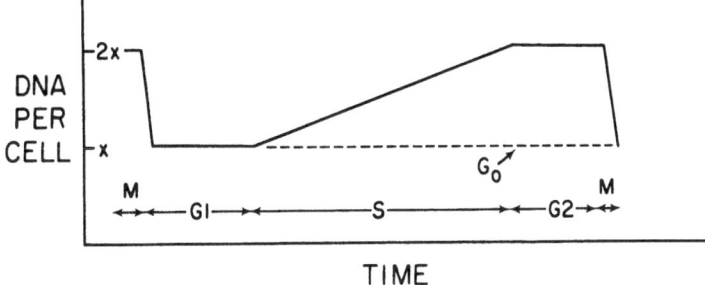

TIME

FIG. 3.8. Phases of DNA synthesis. The normal diploid complement of DNA per cell is assigned the value x. S, G2, and M are fairly constant in duration; G1 is more variable.

In the metamyelocyte compartment, there was no immediate labeling because these are nondividing cells, but after an interval of about 3 hr, labeled metamyelocytes accumulated at 3%/hr. The proportions of meta-myelocytes:juveniles:segmented neutrophils were 1:2.07:2.1. Thus, the average times in each of these compartments would be 33, 69, and 69 hr, and the myelocyte-to-blood time would be 7 days.

This last figure is, of course, testable by seeing when labeled neutrophils do in fact appear in the blood. In various patients, values of 48–144 hr (2–6 days) were found. The low values were found exclusively in the presence of severe infection, and it was thought that they reflected an accelerated flow of neutrophils through the precursor stages into the blood. The usual values were 5–6 days, or distinctly less than the 7-day estimate given above. This difference was thought to be due to departures from strict "pipeline" kinetics, in that once a cell had reached the mature stage, it had an appreciable chance of entering the bloodstream without waiting any longer. A method depending on the first appearance of labeled cells would therefore underestimate the *average* marrow residence time.

The emergence time for band cells was 24 hr less than that for segmented cells, confirming that bands are younger forms. However, the emergence times for cells with 2–5 nuclear segments were identical, a finding that contradicts the commonly held belief that hypersegmented cells are older.

(b) FLM Method. The fraction labeled mitoses method depends upon flash-labeling the cells under study with tritiated thymidine and determining the percentage of mitosing cells that are labeled at short intervals thereafter. In theory, all the labeled cells should go into mitosis synchronously, and at this point, all mitoses are labeled. Later on, only cells that were not in the S phase at the time of labeling will be in mitosis, and no mitoses are

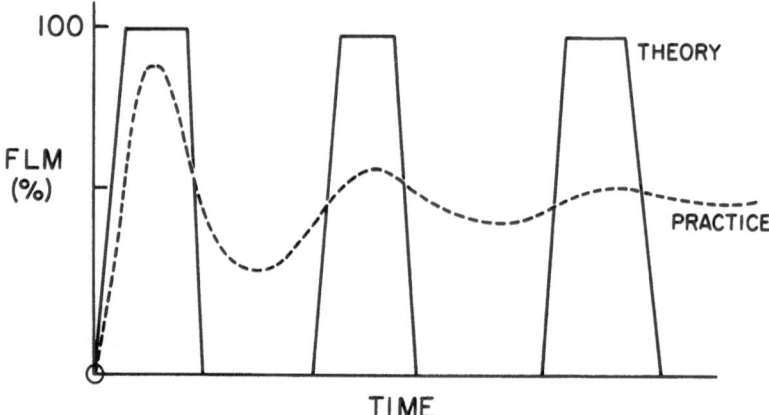

FIG. 3.9. The fraction labeled mitoses method. In theory, the count should oscillate from 0 to
100% indefinitely; in practice, randomization occurs within one or two cycles.

labeled. If the cell cycles remain synchronous, the fraction of labeled
mitoses will regularly oscillate between 0 and 100%, and the wave interval
represents the generation time (Fig. 3.9). Unfortunately, even in uniform
tissue, asynchrony develops quickly, and only one or two cycles are
observed. Various sophisticated methods of treating the data to obtain
more cycles are available, but suffer from the usual problem of whether the
mathematics, however intellectually satisfying, is really representative of
the biological process.[7]

(c) Double Label Technique. The third method involves a double
labeling of the tissue with both tritiated thymidine and ^{14}C-labeled thymidine.[8] The ^{3}H-labeled thymidine is given first, the ^{14}C-labeled thymidine
after an interval that should be no greater than $G2 + \frac{1}{2}M$, and in practice is
usually 1 hr. During this time, some cells that were in the S phase and took
up the ^{3}H label will have moved on to the $G2$ phase, and will not take up the
^{14}C label. About 15 min after the ^{14}C label is given, marrow smears are
made and coated with two layers of photographic emulsion, separated by a
layer of celloidin. The electrons emitted when tritium decays are of very
low energy ($E_{max} = 0.018$ MeV), and are unable to penetrate the celloidin
layer, or to travel any distance laterally. A nucleus containing tritium
therefore gives rise to silver grains that are found only in the first emulsion
layer, and are strictly localized over the nucleus. A nucleus containing ^{14}C,
the decay electrons of which have more energy ($E_{max} = 0.155$ MeV), gives
rise to a "spray" of grains that surround the cell and are found in both
emulsion layers. With this technique, it is possible to distinguish cells

labeled with ^{3}H only from those labeled with ^{14}C. Many of the latter cells, of course, will also contain the ^{3}H label, but these cannot be distinguished with certainty from cells that entered the S phase after tritiated thymidine was given, and therefore contain only ^{14}C label. The calculations go as follows:

The proportion of cells labeled with ^{14}C (with or without ^{3}H) is clearly equal to the ratio between T_s and the generation time T_G:

$$\text{L.I.}_{^{14}\text{C}} = \frac{T_s}{T_G}$$

The proportion of cells that take up ^{3}H is, of course, identical; however, only those that leave the S phase before the ^{14}C label is given will be recognized. If the interval between the labels is T, then the proportion of ^{3}H-labeled cells that leave the S phase is T/T_S.

Thus,

$$\text{L.I.}_{^3\text{H}} = \frac{T_S}{T_G} \cdot \frac{T}{T_S} = \frac{T}{T_G}$$

Therefore,

$$\frac{\text{L.I.}_{^3\text{H}}}{\text{L.I.}_{^{14}\text{C}}} = \frac{T/T_G}{T_s/T_G} = \frac{T}{T_s}$$

or

$$T_s = \frac{\text{L.I.}_{^{14}\text{C}}}{\text{L.I.}_{^3\text{H}}} \cdot T$$

and from this T_G can be calculated.

3.2.3. Critique of Marrow Kinetic Methods

It is unfortunate that bone marrow is so complex a tissue that the application of the fraction labeled mitoses method, the double label method, and other methods not discussed here has given rise to a great deal of controversy and relatively few agreed facts. In the first place, all the elementary calculations presented so far ignore the variations in T_m, T_G, and T_s among different cell populations. All the equations must be corrected for the proportion (usually unknown) of nondividing, or G_0, cells. There are immense practical difficulties in determining just what group a cell belongs to, and what the precise proportions of various groups are. Cells are particularly difficult to identify when they are in mitosis, for nuclear morphology is lost as a diagnostic character. All these considerations combine to produce a situation in which estimates of generation time, compartment transit time, and number of mitoses per compartment are subject to very large errors, and to make matters worse, there is usually no way of estimating just how big the errors are likely to be. There is no better example of the present state of confusion than the question of ineffective granulopoiesis.

3.2.4. Ineffective Granulopoiesis?

Since 1958, Patt and Maloney have maintained that a very substantial number of myelocytes die or are otherwise removed from the marrow before they can mature into metamyelocytes. They proposed originally that as many as 60% of myelocytes might so die, and in their latest paper, in 1971, they still insist that the proportion cannot be less than 40%.[9] The original papers were based on grain count halving times, but as each new technique has become available, they have used it in their beagles and have come up with the same T_s (5 hr) and the same proportion of myelocyte loss. Their latest paper examines the relative rates of release of erythrocytes and neutrophils to the bloodstream. The labeling indices and the T_s and T_G estimates were equal for erythrocyte and neutrophil precursors, and it is agreed by many workers that roughly equal numbers of each cell type are released to the blood each day. But the proportion of neutrophil precursors in marrow smears is twice that of erythroid precursors; ergo, ineffective granulopoiesis must be occurring.

No one else in the field wants to believe this. Bone marrow is in aggregate one of the largest organs in the body, and it is inherently improbable that such huge numbers of cells would die routinely throughout life. In any rapidly dividing cell population, a proportion of the individuals produced are defective and are destroyed, but this proportion is of the order of 5%, not 50%. In the thymus, over 90% of cells produced die without ever leaving the organ, but it is thought that these represent "forbidden clones" of cells that would be dangerous to the body if they were released, and their destruction is thus purposive. Furthermore, there is not the slightest morphological evidence to suggest that such a process goes on in bone marrow; pyknotic myelocytes are infrequent, and karyor-rhexis or phagocytosis of myelocytes is not seen. The universal reaction is to doubt the evidence on which the conclusion is based, and yet no one has convincingly refuted it. The experiments are internally consistent, and, as mentioned, the same answer was obtained by at least five different methods. Their estimate for T_s is considerably shorter than that obtained by most workers, and many feel that here is the error that leads to an underestimate of generation time and an inflation of the estimated birthrate in the myelocyte compartment. Probably, the present answer must be that the available methods are too imprecise to allow a resolution of the question. At any rate, Constable and Blackett recently attempted to settle the problem using the fraction labeled mitoses method with computer analysis of the data.[10] They concluded that the range of variation was such that they were unable to distinguish between no myelocyte loss and 50% myelocyte loss, and that they were unable to decide another perennial question: whether myelocytes are to any degree self-renewing.

3.2.5. DFP Methods

Although the evidence from DNA labels leaves the details of neutro-phil production somewhat obscure, the main outlines of the system are confirmed by experiments using a completely different label, diisopropyl-fluoro[32] phosphate (DFP). This compound binds covalently to the serine hydroxyl groups of certain proteins found in cell membranes. Labeling occurs spontaneously when drug and cells are incubated together under physiological conditions of temperature and pH, and the labeled cells show no discernible functional impairment. Since ^{32}P has a short half-life (14 days), and the decay electron has a relatively high energy ($E_{max} = 1.7$ MeV), the cells are very "hot," and there are few counting problems. The label does not elute from the cells, and when the cell dies and is broken down into its building blocks, the DFP serine cannot be reused for protein synthesis. DFP is fairly specific for neutrophils and their precursors when used in the correct dose; red cells and platelets are labeled much less heavily, and simple methods for separating neutrophils from other blood cells can be used without much error. The method is quite useless for obtaining information about individual cells because ^{32}P decay electrons are too energetic to give good resolution in autoradiograms; however, such information can be obtained from supplemental experiments with ^3H-labeled DFP.

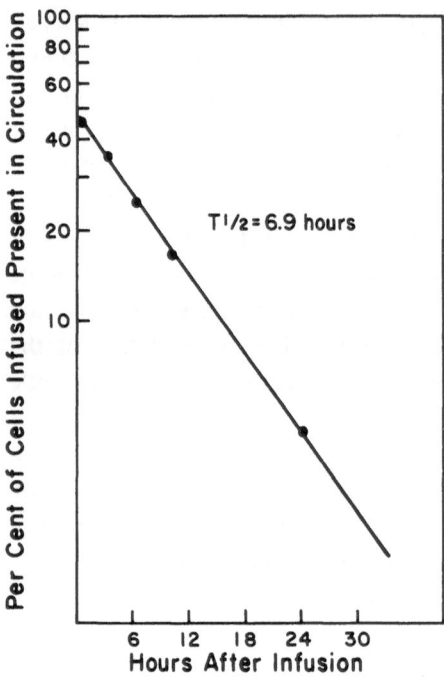

FIG. 3.10. Blood granulocyte radio-activity in normal man infused with DF³²P-labeled granulocytes. [From Cartwright *et al.*, *Blood* **24**:780 (1964),[11] by permission.]

The simplest type of experiment is to withdraw 500 ml of blood from a normal man into a plastic bag containing heparin and DF³²P.[11] The blood is incubated for 1 hr, at the end of which time the DFP has bound to cells or to plasma proteins, or has been hydrolyzed by the fluorophosphatases that abound in normal tissue and serum. A sample of blood is removed for determination of the initial leukocyte radioactivity, and the rest is rein-fused. At intervals thereafter, blood samples are withdrawn, the leukocytes are isolated, and the specific radioactivity (cpm/mg protein) determined. These counts are essentially all in neutrophils, as was demonstrated by experiments with ³H-labeled DFP that showed no uptake by lymphocytes, basophils, or eosinophils, and only trivial uptake by monocytes.

The results of this experiment are shown in Fig. 3.10. The blood neutrophil radioactivity declines exponentially, and at least up to 30 hr, the exponential has only one component. The half-life is about 7 hr, and when the line is extrapolated back to zero time, the intercept is always less than 100%, usually about 50%. This last finding would suggest that about half the labeled neutrophils are so badly damaged that they are immediately removed from the bloodstream by reticuloendothelial cells. However, this is probably not the explanation, because if the recipient is given epinephrine or is vigorously exercised immediately after infusion, the extrapolated initial concentration rises sharply, occasionally to as much as 100%. It has long been known that neutrophils tend to travel in the peripheral layers of blood in the small vessels, and that they frequently attach temporarily to the endothelium and subsequently release their hold. It is difficult to quantitate this process, or indeed to be certain that the thin tissue preparations in which it is seen are in their normal state. Nevertheless, it is proposed that the neutrophils that cannot be accounted for are mostly stuck reversibly to the walls of small vessels, and that blood neutrophils can be divided into two pools, a circulating granulocyte pool (C.G.P.) and a marginated granulocyte pool (M.G.P.). Cells pass from one pool to the other so rapidly that equilibration is complete within minutes of reinjection of the labeled blood. Exercise and epinephrine reduce the tendency of neutrophils to stick to vessel walls, and cause more of the injected cells to be demonstrable in the circulating pool.

That the decay curve is a simple exponential means that cells must leave the circulation by a random process that is not related to their age. To see why this is so, consider the curve that would be obtained if neutrophils had a fixed average lifetime of 30 hr and assume that a cell was removed at the end of that time. The blood removed for labeling would contain cells of different ages; on average, $\frac{1}{30}$th would be 30 hr old, $\frac{1}{30}$th would be 29 hr, and so on. When the labeled cells were reinfused, $\frac{1}{30}$th would be removed in the first hour, $\frac{1}{30}$th in the second hour, and there would be a linear drop in radioactivity with respect to time. What is actually observed is that a constant fraction of the cells in the blood is removed in unit time, and that fraction remains constant for as long as there is enough radioactivity to measure. Therefore, if there is an upper limit to a neutrophil's life span, less than 1% of cells remain in the bloodstream long enough to reach it.

Actually, Cronkite suggested on the basis of radioautographic data that a small fraction of blood neutrophils might reach their biological life span and then be subject to rapid removal.[12] In smears of normal blood, 0.02–0.1% of neutrophils show pyknotic nuclei, usually regarded as a sign of cell death. In patients given tritiated thymidine, label first appears in these pyknotic cells about 30 hr after the first labeled neutrophils appear in the bloodstream. Given a half-life of 7 hr for neutrophils, the proportion of pyknotic cells should therefore be at least $\frac{1}{32}$ (35 hr = 5 half-lives, so the proportion should be greater than $[\frac{1}{2}]^5$). Given the very small proportion actually observed, Cronkite calculated that the half-life of senescent cells must be about 15 min. This conclusion seems eminently reasonable, but the fact remains that the overwhelming majority of neutrophils leave by the random process demonstrated by the $DF^{32}P$ data. The estimate of a 30-hr absolute limit may be too short, because there is evidence that transfused neutrophils (marked by the Pelger–Hüet anomaly) may persist in the circulation for as long as 50 hr. Also, some $DF^{32}P$ experiments have been carried out to 4 days without seeing evidence of accelerated loss of cells.

Other inferences that may be drawn from the exponential removal of neutrophils are that once cells have left the bone marrow, they do not return in significant numbers; and similarly, once they have left the bloodstream, they do not reenter it. Neither of these processes would be compatible with a simple exponential, and furthermore, there is abundant evidence from studies with DNA labels that neutrophils travel on a one-way street. To cite one example, Perry gave ^{32}P to dogs and waited until the blood radioactivity was declining because most of the labeled cells had entered the tissues.[13] Neutrophil leukocytosis was then induced by injecting typhoid vaccine, but in all cases, only unlabeled cells from bone marrow were found in the blood, and there was no evidence of return of neutrophils from the tissues.

DFP can also be given intravenously, and under these circumstances, neutrophil precursors in bone marrow, as well as circulating cells, become labeled. The extent to which various types of cells become labeled was investigated using [^{3}H]DFP and autoradiography. In round figures, myelocytes became labeled to about 50% of the level seen in the circulating granulocytes, and metamyelocytes, band cells, juveniles, and mature forms all became labeled to about 25% of the circulating level. Promyelocytes and myeloblasts did not label at all.

Fortuitously, these labeling indices combined to give a rather simple curve for the radioactivity of blood neutrophils after $DF^{32}P$ had been given intravenously. This curve fell into three parts (Fig. 3.11). In the first part, neutrophil radioactivity declined with a half-life of 7 hr to a level of 25% of the initial labeling. This decline represented elimination of those neutrophils that became labeled in the circulating blood. Then there was a plateau period, during which blood neutrophils were produced by maturation of the metamyelocytes and other nondividing members of the bone marrow pool that had been labeled at 25% of the initial blood level. At the end of the plateau, cells were being produced that were the descendants of the myelocytes that had been labeled with 50% efficiency; however, these cells

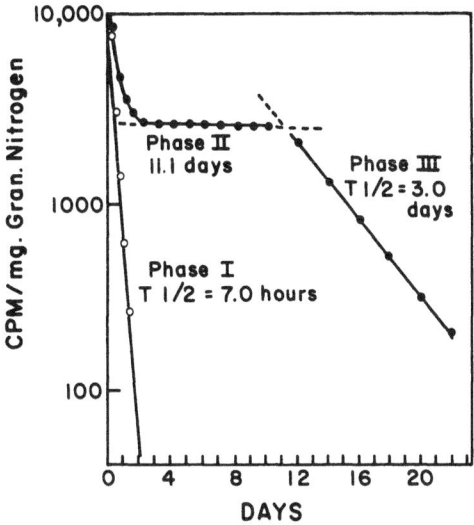

FIG. 3.11.   Blood granulocyte radioactivity in normal man infused with DF³²P intravenously.
(From Cartwright et al,[11] by permission.)

had divided once, and accordingly, the 25% plateau continued for a total
duration of about 11 days. In the third phase, there was a slow exponential
decline with a half-life of 2.9 days, and by 24 days after the injection,
granulocyte radioactivity was at background levels. It was thought that the
final decline represented dilution by successive mitoses of label originally
taken up by myelocytes.

The evidence obtained by the use of DF³²P pertains mainly to the
mature neutrophils in the circulating blood and to the nondividing pool of
precursors in the marrow. Information from DF³²P therefore complements
the evidence from DNA labels very satisfactorily. The *in vitro* method is
subject to considerable random error (due to factors such as errors in
differential counts), and there is in addition a systematic error due to the
fact that a few cells are irreversibly damaged by the labeling procedure and
are removed from the circulation soon after reinfusion. These errors lead to
an overestimate of the total blood granulocyte pool. Despite these errors, it
is clear that normal men show very considerable variations in the size of
the total pool, and in the proportion of neutrophils marginated at any one
time (Table 3.2). These variations occur among subjects, and also in the
same subject from time to time.

TABLE 3.2. Granulocyte Kinetics in Normal Man

(Data obtained by the $DF^{32}P$ technique. From Cartwright et al.[11])

Parameter	Number of subjects	Mean	95% limits
Total blood granulocyte pool			
$\times\ 10^7$ cells/kg	109	70	14–160
Circulating pool $\times\ 10^7$ cells/kg	109	31	11–46
Marginated pool $\times\ 10^7$ cells/kg	109	39	0–85
Half-life (hr)	56	6.7	4–10
Granulocyte turnover rate $\times$			
10^7 cells/kg per day	56	163	50–340

3.3. Neutrophil Precursors Which Cannot Be Recognized Morphologically

3.3.1. The Hemopoietic Stem Cell

So far in this chapter, we have been concerned with the production of mature neutrophils from marrow cells that have been traced back to the myeloblast level. It is not known to what extent the myeloblast pool normally reproduces itself, but it is clear that when the demand for neutrophils is great, the myeloblast pool can be augmented by an input from pools of less differentiated cells. It is not possible to identify these cells morphologically, but in the last fifteen years, some fascinating physiological evidence has been obtained that gives an idea of the potentialities of the system.

Most of the available information has come from experiments on lethally irradiated mice. Radiation damages all the tissues of the body, but it is especially lethal to rapidly dividing cells. In a whole animal, the most susceptible cells are those in the bone marrow and in the epithelia of the gastrointestinal tract. It so happens that bone marrow is irreversibly damaged by about half the level of radiation required for gastrointestinal epithelium, and a dose of radiation can be found that produces fairly pure bone marrow failure. A mouse so irradiated develops agranulocytosis in the course of a week or two and dies of overwhelming infection. It can be rescued by giving it an injection of bone marrow cells from a normal mouse of the same genotype.

The mechanism by which this process occurs was studied in a classic paper by Becker, McCulloch, and Till.[14] They irradiated mice, reconstituted them with very small doses of bone marrow cells, and examined the spleens at various intervals after irradiation. They found that if the dose was small enough, foci ("colonies") of hemopoietic tissue developed that were completely separated from each other and could be counted. The number of foci found was directly proportional to the dose of cells injected, which suggested that each colony originated from a single cell of the initial inoculum. (If two, three . . . cells had to cooperate to found a colony, then the number of colonies would be proportional to the square, cube . . . of the number of cells injected.) However, since it was possible that small clumps of cells existed in the initial inoculum and that the required cell associations were already established, further evidence was sought by irradiating the donor marrow cells before they were transfused into the irradiated recipient.

Radiation may produce chromosome abnormalities that can be seen morphologically when a stained squash preparation of a mitosing cell is examined. Some of the abnormalities are so gross that the cell cannot reproduce, but others do allow cell division, and the abnormal chromosomes are faithfully duplicated and passed on to the daughter cells. Since the chromosome abnormality in any one irradiated cell is unique, all the descendants of that cell carry a label by which they can be identified.

Becker, McCulloch, and Till examined the mitoses seen in individual spleen colonies and asked the question, "Do all mitoses in this colony show the *same* abnormal karyotype?" In most colonies, all the cells showed no recognizable abnormality, but a few were seen that did, and in all such cases, over 95% of the mitosing cells in the colony showed the same karyotypic abnormality.

When the cells in individual colonies were examined cytologically, it was found that some were composed of erythrocyte precursors, some contained granulocytes, and some contained megakaryocytes and platelets. Some colonies were mixed, and contained more than one cell line, the most common example being simultaneous production of neutrophils and platelets. Mixed colonies also contained identical abnormal karyotypes in all cells.

Because of these results, it was proposed that there existed a "stem cell" capable of differentiating into any of the cell lines found in normal bone marrow. This hypothesis has since been abundantly confirmed. Perhaps the most cogent evidence was obtained by Trentin and his colleagues, who irradiated mice, injected them with small numbers of bone marrow cells, and removed the spleens at a stage where colonies were visible and clearly separated.[15] It was known that if the cells of any one colony were transferred to another irradiated mouse, all cellular types of colonies were found in this second mouse, indicating that some of the cells in each colony retained their primitive multipotentiality. The number of stem cells in one colony was insufficient to reconstitute an irradiated recipient, so a series of *in vivo* multiplications was used. Cells from one colony, the offspring of one stem cell, were transferred to an irradiated recipient. From the spleen of this recipient, daughter colonies were obtained and transferred to several irradiated mice. From these mice, colonies were transferred to 20 or 30 irradiated mice, and the colonies that now developed were sufficient to reconstitute a single irradiated recipient with enough cells to allow him to recover and survive for an extended period. The bone marrow, blood, and lymphoid organs of such a mouse were morphologically normal, and it was shown that the immune system was capable of mounting antibody responses against several diverse antigens. Since all the bone marrow and lymphoid cells in this mouse originated from a single cell, the hypothesis that stem cells are multipotent seems proved.

The direction in which a stem cell differentiates is influenced by the milieu in which it finds itself. Thus, if the irradiated recipient is transfused with enough erythrocytes to raise the hematocrit to 70%, then fewer spleen colonies are composed of erythrocyte precursors. Conversely, if the recipient is anemic, erythroid colonies not only are more frequent, but also are larger and contain more cells. Also, stem cells that lodge in the spleen make a high proportion of erythroid colonies, whereas those in the bone marrow are more likely to develop into myeloid cells.

It is clear that stem cells cannot give rise directly to myeloblasts, or to erythroblasts either. Bone marrow contains only about 20 stem cells/10,000 nucleated cells, or 0.2%. Myeloblasts constitute 2% of bone marrow cells and have a compartment transit time of about 24 hr. If such a pool were renewed directly from the stem cell level, the stem cells would have to have a generation time of about 2 hr, even if no allowance is made for the demands of erythropoiesis. No mammalian cell can divide at such a rate, and indeed there is substantial evidence that under normal circumstances, most of the stem cell population is not dividing at all. This evidence is based on the "thymidine suicide," technique in which a mouse is injected with a very large dose of ^{3}H thymidine. Any cell in the S phase takes up so much radioactive label that it is killed, and because of the low energy level of tritium decay electrons, surrounding cells are unharmed. This procedure leads to only a slight fall in the number of stem cells, as measured by the colony counting technique.[16]

There must therefore be some kind of cell ancestral to the myeloblast, and descended from the stem cell. It seems likely from several lines of evidence that these cells are more restricted in their capability for differentiation than are the stem cells. Thus, in chronic myelocytic leukemia, a pathognomonic abnormal chromosome, the Philadelphia chromosome, is found not only in neutrophil precursors, but also in megakaryocytes and erythroblasts. However, the overwhelming majority of investigators have not found it in lymphocytes. If mice are transfused to raise the hematocrit to 60–70%, the spontaneous production of erythrocytes essentially ceases. Injection of the hormone erythropoietin produces a sudden increase of pronormoblasts, which synthesize hemoglobin and eventually mature into erythrocytes. The "erythropoietin-sensitive cells" that differentiate into pronormoblasts are severely depleted by the thymidine suicide technique described above. This finding suggests that, unlike stem cells, they are in continous cell cycle. This sort of evidence would suggest that there is a hierarchy of cells, the potentialities of which become progressively more restricted until they are committed to the production of one cell line, and respond selectively to the hormones that promote differentiation along that line. In the case of the neutrophil, one of these partially committed ancestral cells is probably exemplified by the colony forming cell.

3.3.2. The Colony-Forming Cell

If bone marrow cells are suspended in tissue culture medium and plated out in a semisolid medium of methyl cellulose or agar, some of the cells may proliferate and form small colonies. This proliferation takes place only in the presence of a glycoprotein, the colony-stimulating factor (CSF). Originally, the CSF was supplied by a "feeder" layer of cells incorporated in an 0.5% agar layer underneath the semisolid layer in which the marrow cells were to grow.[17] Now it is usually prepared from human urine, from serum, or by using the tissue culture medium from suitable cells. Obviously, soluble CSF is preferable to the cumbersome feeder layer method.

The colonies that develop are composed mostly of neutrophils and their precursors at first, but even early on, there are colonies of pure monocytes and macrophages and mixed colonies containing both cell lines.

As time goes on, macrophage colonies come to predominate, apparently because the cells that originally gave rise to neutrophil precursors change their direction of differentiation.[18]

The number of colony-forming cells (CFCs) in bone marrow is usually about 1 per 100 plated cells, and because of this ratio, it could not be assumed that one colony arises from a single cell. However, Moore and his colleagues were able to fractionate monkey bone marrow on albumin gradients and obtain suspensions of cells of which up to 25% were CFCs.[19] From these fractions, individual cells could be transferred to culture medium and the development of colonies observed directly. The colonies were typical of those formed from suspensions of whole bone marrow, including the early granulocytic predominance and the subsequent shift to macrophage production.

The colony forming cell looked like a rather large lymphocyte, with scanty cytoplasm and no granules. There is now much disagreement about whether the colony forming cell can be defined in morphological terms; McCullough has consistently found that cells that operationally are colony forming cells may vary substantially in size, appearance, and density. Parenthetically, it may be added that attempts have been made to identify the multipotential hemopoietic stem cell with an unusual type of cell that vaguely resembles a lymphocyte,[20] and again McCullough denies that operationally defined stem cells have a constant morphological appearance.

3.4. Summary

Neutrophils arise ultimately from stem cells in bone marrow that are capable of differentiating into erythrocyte, lymphocyte, monocyte, and megakaryocyte precursors, as well as neutrophil precursors. Under normal circumstances, stem cells are mostly resting, but they can be stimulated into activity by a sudden demand for any of the bone marrow cell lines. Most of the self-renewing mitotic activity required to supply the neutrophil compartment of bone marrow probably goes on in an intermediate population of cells with more restricted potentialities. It is likely that there is more than one type of such cell, but our knowledge of these early stages is fragmentary, and we have virtually no quantitative data about cell numbers or kinetics. It seems that once a cell has differentiated to the myeloblast stage, it is committed to the neutrophil line and is no longer capable of true self-regenerating activity.

At this stage, we are able to apply numbers, albeit with large error coefficients, to the cell populations and transit times. Maturation from myeloblast to mature neutrophil typically takes from four to seven cell divisions, and occupies a period of between 1 and 2 weeks. Some cells may persist at the myelocyte stage for extended periods of time, either by entering a G_0 phase or possibly by a limited number of self-renewing divisions. The idea that some cells can escape from strict pipeline kinetics, at least for a time, would account for the uncertainties about whether or not a large fraction of myelocytes die before maturity. The final product of these successive stages of maturation is the marrow granulocyte reserve of juvenile and mature polymorphs. These cells amount to about half of all the cells in bone marrow, and are released to the blood in huge numbers, about 1.12×10^{11} mature neutrophils per day in a 70-kg man. If neutrophils were a discrete organ, it would be growing at the rate of between 50 and 100 g/day. However, the half-life of neutrophils in blood is very short, only about 7 hr. Where the cells go, what they may do, and how the whole system is controlled will be taken up in the next chapter.

Selected Reading

LoBue, J., Stem cell and neutrophilic granulocyte kinetics, *Med. Clin. North Am.* 57:265 (1973).

Metcalf, D., and Moore, M. A. S., *Haemopoietic Cells,* American Elsevier Publishing Co., New York, 1971.

Haemopoietic Stem Cells, Ciba Foundation Symposium 13 (new series), Associated Scientific Publishers, Amsterdam, 1973.

4

Tissue Consumption of Granulocytes and Control Mechanisms for Granulopoiesis

The reader in search of hard scientific information would do well to skip this chapter altogether, because it is constructed from a few wattles of established fact and large quantities of speculative daub. It was shown in the last chapter that enormous numbers of neutrophils are produced in the marrow, enter the bloodstream, and rapidly leave the blood for the tissues. Intuitively, one would suppose that their function was to combat bacterial infections, and that the cells would emigrate chiefly from blood vessels in those areas of the body where large bacterial populations are normally carried. If this were so, there should be heavy emigration of labeled neutrophils into the mouth, the gastrointestinal tract, the upper airway, and perhaps the skin, and very little into normally sterile areas, such as the brain and skeletal muscle. How far does the available evidence support this picture?

4.1. Distribution, Function, and Disposal of Neutrophils

Histologically, it can be shown that small numbers of neutrophils (and eosinophils) are normally found infiltrating the mucous membranes of the

gastrointestinal tract and the upper airway, and under the stratified squa-
mous epithelia of the skin, esophagus, and vagina. In germ-free animals,
these infiltrates are less prominent. Godwin *et al.* showed that rats raised
with special precautions to avoid the common laboratory epidemic diseases
("specific pathogen-free rats") had blood neutrophil counts that were about
60% of those found in conventional rats.[1] Fliedner *et al.* gave tritiated
thymidine to germ-free mice and measured the time that elapsed until the
blood neutrophils were maximally labeled.[2] This time is a rough measure of
the maturation time from myelocyte to polymorph, and proved to be about
92 hr, as against 82 hr for a conventional mouse. The life span of neutrophils in the blood was unaltered. An extensive study of germ-free mice was
conducted by Boggs and his colleagues.[3] They counted neutrophil precursors in bone marrow and were unable to find any significant differences
from the normal. They confirmed that the blood neutrophil count was
significantly lower. When germ-free mice were moved to a conventional
environment, there was a sudden depletion of the mature neutrophil pool in
the bone marrow, well marked at 16 hr, and during the next month, there
was evidence of increase in the mitotic compartment. By 3 months, the
marrow was back to normal. Overall, the differences between germ-free
and conventional animals seem relatively minor, and it is difficult to see
how bacteria can greatly affect the distribution of neutrophils under ordinary circumstances.

In man, fairly large numbers of neutrophils can be collected from
saliva, or by washing out the normal mouth with saline. If labeled neutrophils are circulating, the specific radioactivity of mouth leukocytes mirrors
that of the blood. Other known routes for external loss of neutrophils are
the urine (up to 2×10^5 cells/hr) and the secretions of the *cervix uteri* during
the second half of the menstrual cycle. Neutrophils are not normally found
in nasal or bronchial secretions, and their presence here is regarded as
presumptive evidence of infection. None of these routes can account for
more than a tiny fraction of the known neutrophil turnover, although it
might be enlightening to have figures for neutrophil emigration into the
bowel.

If neutrophils are not lost by external migration, they must be disposed
of in the tissues. In tissue culture, neutrophils die within a day or two, and
either disintegrate or are taken up by macrophages if any are present. It is
not easy to examine normal tissue microscopically over long periods of
time. Probably the nearest approach is obtained with the rabbit ear chamber, where a disc of tissue is punched out and discarded, and the hole is

enclosed between two transparent plates. Granulation tissue grows into the space and organizes, and with luck, the preparation can be examined over periods of many months. The tissue could hardly be described as normal, and is more likely in a state of low-grade inflammation; however, neutrophils may be observed to crawl about for 3 or 4 days, then die and disintegrate. It has been suggested that the dissolution of neutrophils in normal tissue may subserve a nutritive function for that tissue. This idea has a suspicious history, because until we recently became aware of what lymphocytes actually do, this was thought to be their function. The alleged process was even given an appropriately scientific-sounding name, and the cells were said to be *trephocytic*.

A more likely function for neutrophils in tissue is to deal with foreign material, both living and dead, that succeeds in crossing the mechanical barriers between the tissues and the outside world. It seems probable that small numbers of bacteria frequently penetrate the nasal or intestinal mucosa, and that they are disposed of without causing noticeable local inflammatory changes.[4] Furthermore, antigens in food, in inspired particles, and from local commensal bacterial populations are known to frequently enter tissue and initiate immunological reactions of various sorts. Neutrophils are powerfully attracted by antigen–antibody complexes, and chemotactic factors are generated during both immediate and delayed hypersensitivity reactions. If significant numbers of neutrophils are in fact consumed by responding to antigens, this consumption would explain why the turnovers in germ-free (but not antigen-free) animals are not greatly different from the normal. It would also fit in with the evidence that significant numbers of neutrophils enter lymph nodes (see below). Last, it is possible that neutrophils play a role in the disposal of dead and dying tissue cells.

Tissue culture and rabbit ear chamber results would suggest that neutrophils entering tissue will die and disintegrate there in a fairly short time. They provide no information about how important is entry into solid tissue, as opposed to external loss.

Nearly twenty years ago, Julian and Clara Ambrus investigated this problem by the techniques that were then available, and while their experiments can be severely criticized, they are worth discussing.[5] The first type of experiment was to pass polyethylene catheters into the arteries and veins of various organs in the dog, and count the number of cells entering and leaving. Most of these experiments involved the use of barbiturate anesthesia, but in the case of the lung, some experiments were done in chronic preparations without anesthesia. It was found that neutrophils were selectively removed from the arterial blood by the lungs, the liver, and the spleen.

Confirmatory evidence was obtained by perfusing isolated dog organs *in vitro*. The liver appeared to "regulate" the concentration of neutrophils in the blood used to perfuse it, cells being removed until the concentration was about $1000/mm^3$. Repeated perfusions with the same blood led to no more removal of neutrophils, but when new blood was used, the concentration was rapidly reduced to the same level. Experiments with spleen produced similar results, although as Barcroft showed long ago, the dog spleen contains very large numbers of sequestered neutrophils, and any stimulation of its sympathetic nervous supply leads to splenic contraction and the expulsion of neutrophils into the splenic veins. The lungs were found to regulate the granulocyte count of the blood even more efficiently than the liver, only about 3 min being required to reduce the granulocyte count to the steady-state value of about $1000/mm^3$. If new blood was introduced, the neutrophil count was rapidly reduced, and this procedure could be repeated many times.

Even more interesting, if blood from which the neutrophils had been removed was used, the lungs released neutrophils to bring the concentration up to the steady-state level. This latter result suggested that neutrophils were reversibly marginated on capillary walls (see Chapter 3). However, the lungs were able to remove neutrophils at the same rate when new blood was added every 5–10 min over a 6-hr period, whereas their capacity to restore neutrophils to the blood was exhausted after three changes. A large majority of the neutrophils were clearly migrating into the pulmonary tissue.

Since it was possible that all tissues subjected to grossly unphysiological procedures would remove granulocytes from the blood, they studied the isolated dog hind leg. Here, there was no difference in the neutrophil content of arterial and venous blood, which presumably is evidence that skin, bone, and skeletal muscle do not account for much of the normal consumption of neutrophils.

Only primitive neutrophil labels were available in 1957: quinacrine, a fluorescent dye that bound to neutrophils and seriously depressed their respiration, and ^{32}P introduced by injecting radioactive phosphate into a suitable donor animal and recovering labeled cells from the blood several days later. It was found that there was heavy migration of labeled cells into the tracheobronchial tree, from which they could be recovered by washing out the lungs with saline. If the animal was allowed to survive, the cells apparently migrated up the trachea and were swallowed.

The migration of neutrophils into the gastrointestinal tract was studied in dogs who had surgically created openings into the esophagus, stomach, or small bowel. They were studied after all incisions had healed and they were gaining weight. Substantial numbers of neutrophils were recovered from the esophagus and stomach, and lesser numbers from the small bowel. The large bowel was not studied.

The accumulation of neutrophils in solid tissues was studied by determining the concentrations of ^{32}P the tissues contained after injection of labeled cells. ^{32}P was present in several forms, which were measured separately: DNA, RNA, phospholipid, phosphoprotein, organic acid–soluble phosphates (ATP, etc.), and inorganic phosphate. If all these components were present in an organ in the same proportions as those in the injected cells, that was evidence that whole cells were present in the organ, and confirmation was sought with the fluorescent quinacrine label. If only DNA and RNA were found, that was thought to indicate that the neutrophils had disintegrated.

It was found that neutrophils accumulated in the lungs, liver, spleen, lymph nodes, bone marrow, and the intestines. In the liver and spleen, they broke up; in the other organs, they appeared to be intact. Quantitatively, accumulation in solid organs appeared to be much more important than external loss. Even in the intestines, the cells appeared to remain in the wall rather than enter the lumen.

Unfortunately, one cannot accept these experiments at face value. Neutrophils are very delicate cells, and the slightest experimental manipulation causes them to agglutinate. It is impossible to regard cells subjected to multiple centrifugations and procedures such as hypotonic lysis as normal, and it is very suspicious that the observed distribution of labeled cells is virtually that of the reticuloendothelial system. The accumulation of labeled neutrophils in lung was specifically denied by Cronkite, who found most of them migrated into lymph nodes. His experiments in turn can be criticized because his cell populations were not pure, and contained lymphocytes.

No more work has been done on this problem in the last few years. The only acceptable methods would be those that could be used in normal, unanesthetized animals with labeled neutrophil populations that had been subjected to minimal experimental manipulation. The $DF^{32}P$ label appears to meet these criteria, and it would be very interesting to see if data obtained with it agreed with the older results.

4.2. Control of the Blood Neutrophil Level

In health, the neutrophil count in the circulating blood varies remarkably little. In adult humans, the absolute number of neutrophils per cubic millimeter ranges from a minimum of about 1500 to a maximum of about 8000, with a mean of 4400. As was mentioned earlier, the circulating pool of granulocytes is in dynamic equilibrium with a pool of cells that appear to be marginated along the walls of capillaries, and is the same size as the circulating pool, or a little larger. The best evidence, obtained by the $DF^{32}P$ method, would suggest that the size of the total blood granulocyte pool in man shows only a threefold variation, from 0.28 to 0.78 $\times$ 10^9 cells/kg.[6] Superimposed on this basic constancy is an ability to mobilize enormous numbers of neutrophils very quickly in response to stimuli as various as muscular exercise and bacterial infection. How is the very complex process of myelopoiesis controlled so as to permit both constancy and flexibility?

It should be admitted at the outset that we have no idea whether the blood concentration of neutrophils is the controlled variable, or whether some kind of tissue demand takes precedence. If the latter, then presumably individual tissues would each have their own needs, and it would be possible to envision the constant blood neutrophil concentration as the resultant of a large number of separate instructions to the bone marrow. The observed distribution of neutrophil counts in normal man is log normal, which would be compatible with either hypothesis.

Armchair theory would suggest a number of possible ways in which neutrophils might be mobilized. The simplest would be to release marginated cells from capillary walls in tissues that do not themselves require neutrophils. Next, it might be possible to release cells from the very large pool of mature and almost mature granulocytes in the bone marrow. As noted, there is considerable uncertainty about the normal behavior of myelocytes, and a number of mechanisms might be imagined at this level. Mitosis might be speeded up. Cells might be inhibited from entering the G_0 phase, or stimulated to leave it. If cell death is a normal phenomenon, that could be inhibited. An extra cell division at this stage would double the production of mature forms. Alternatively, if fewer cell divisions occurred, mature forms could be produced more quickly at the expense of total numbers. This mechanism is not as unplausible as it sounds. In bacterial infections, time is of the essence, and history has repeatedly shown that 500 troops at the height of a battle are worth more than 10,000 when the battle is already lost (Marengo, 1800). There might be similar effects at the level of the committed precursors of myeloblasts. Last, stem cells might be stimulated to differentiate along the pathway leading to neutrophil production.

There is some evidence for all these effects (Fig. 4.1), although it is not possible to synthesize them into a coherent and logically satisfying control process. There is much less evidence for the negative controls that would also be essential in any balanced system. It is worth noting that the time frames of the effects produced by stimulation at various levels are very different. Mobilization of neutrophils from the marrow pool could occur within minutes, and certainly within hours. An effect at the stem cell level would take at least a week to affect delivery of neutrophils to the tissues.

4.2.1. Mobilization from Capillary Walls

A number of forms of vigorous muscular exercise, such as running, playing football, childbirth, and epileptic fits, may be associated with neutrophilia in the 20–30,000 cells/mm^3 range. Lesser degrees of neutrophilia can occur in people under mental strain or suffering from anxiety neurosis. The usual explanation is that all these states are associated with the secretion of epinephrine from the adrenal medulla, and that this secretion causes release of neutrophils from the marginal pool. However, since the marginal pool is only the same size as the circulating one, there are simply not enough marginated cells to raise the neutrophil count to 25,000, so many of the cells must come from the marrow. This view is borne out by the fact that immature cells, even myelocytes, may be found in the bloodstream after vigorous exercise.

4.2.2. Mobilization of the Mature Pool from Bone Marrow

There is substantial evidence for the existence of a factor or factors that cause the release of the postmitotic pool of band cells and segmented neutrophils from the bone marrow. The experiments might be summarized as follows: Neutropenia was induced in donor animals by one means or another, and their serum was injected into normal recipient animals. Within an hour or two, the recipients developed elevated neutrophil counts, which were shown to be due to the release of mature cells from the bone marrow.

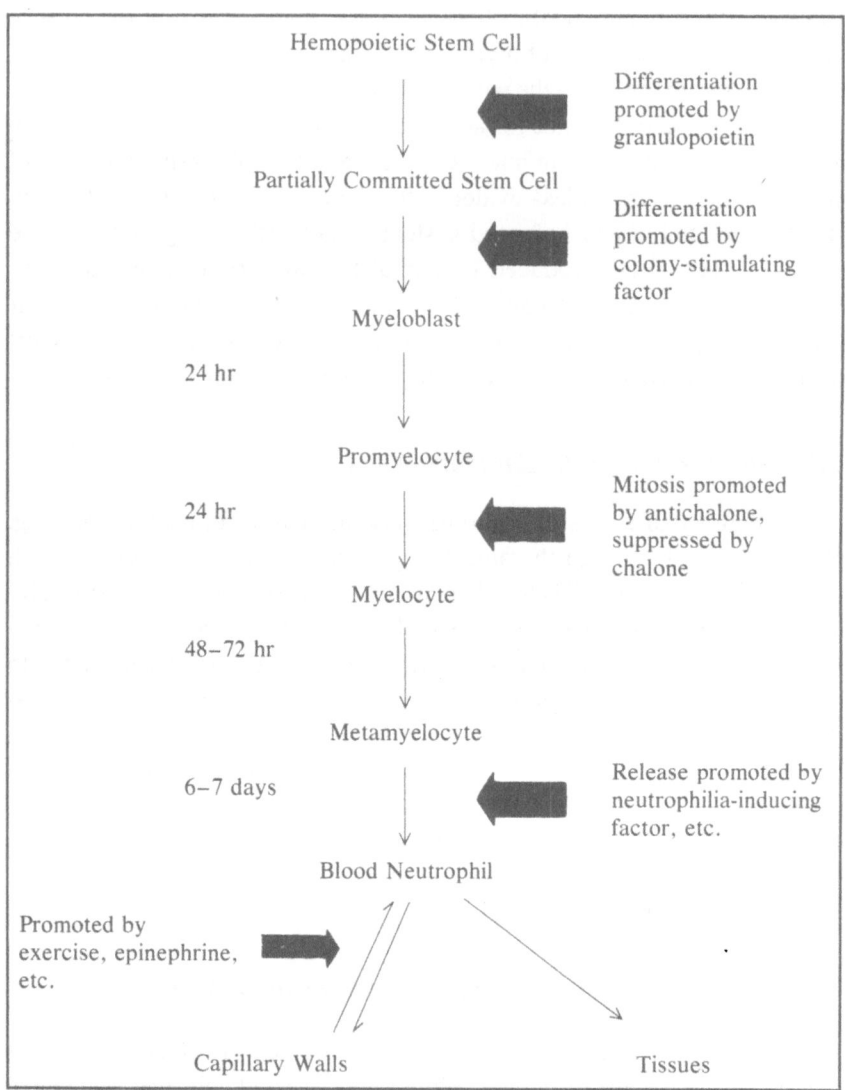

FIG. 4.1. Normal developmental sequence for neutrophils in bone marrow. The sites of action of the putative controlling hormones are indicated.

Injection of serum from normal donors had no such effect. In all these experiments, it was necessary to exclude bacterial infection either of the donor animals or of their serum, because gram-negative bacteria contain in their cell walls an endotoxin that is a powerful inducer of neutrophil leucocytosis. None of the investigators succeeded in precisely characterizing their active material and distinguishing it from endotoxin, but it does seem improbable that the very uniform results observed could all be due to an artifact.

Gordon and his colleagues depleted rats of neutrophils by injecting normal saline solution into the peritoneal cavity.[7] Leukocytes accumulated in the fluid, and if it was drained after 12–18 hr, these leukocytes were lost to the body. After the procedure had been repeated a number of times, serum was taken from these "leukophoresed" rats, and injected into normal rats, which developed a neutrophil leukocytosis maximal at 4–6 hr after injection. Examination of the bone marrow of the recipient rats showed depletion of the band and segmented neutrophils, but not of earlier forms. The liberation of neutrophils from bone marrow was confirmed, using the isolated perfused rat hind leg. Perfusion of the leg with serum from leukophoresed rats led to liberation of neutrophils into the venous effluent, whereas perfusion with normal serum did not.

A more elegant experiment involved uniting two rats in parabiosis. A long incision was made in the left flank of one rat and the right flank of another, from the scapula to the pelvis. The scapulae and pelvic girdles of the two rats were wired together with stainless steel, and the two skin edges were sewed together. After healing, the two rats were united by a broad band of tissue running from shoulder to hip, across which the two circulations communicated. If the right rat were leukophoresed, its neutrophil count fell, and that of the left rat rose. If exudates were induced, but were not drained, the neutrophil counts of both rats remained normal.

These experiments could be explained if loss of neutrophils from the body caused the secretion of a soluble substance that diffused into the blood and, when it reached the bone marrow, stimulated release of neutrophils from the postmitotic pool. Gordon was able to show that the active material behaved like a protein, being nondialyzable, destroyed by heat, and precipitated by ammonium sulfate. Unfortunately, none of these properties excludes the possibility that the effects could be explained by bacterial endotoxin. Endotoxin itself is a lipopolysaccharide, and is strikingly heat-stable. However, in serum it complexes with proteins, and is precipitated along with them by any of the procedures described above.

It is of some interest that Gordon had actually to remove the exudates to stimulate the secretion of his "neutrophilia-inducing factor" (NIF). This necessity would suggest that mere consumption within the body would not be an adequate stimulus, an idea that does not square with results of other investigators using different methods.

Another type of leukophoresis experiment was done by Craddock and his coworkers, who took blood from dogs, centrifuged it, removed the white cells, and returned plasma and red cells to the animal.[8] Dogs so treated developed neutropenia over the first 3 hr, but then the rate of delivery of cells to the blood from the marrow increased, and by 6 hr, it was not possible to keep the neutrophil count depressed, and indeed it often rose above normal despite continued leukophoresis. It was shown that the cells came from the postmitotic pool, because heavily irradiated dogs could still mobilize neutrophils normally until 3 days after the irradiation. Here again, the effective stimulus was a low neutrophil count, since the response could be inhibited by transfusing enough dog granulocytes to keep the blood count normal. The mobilization process could be switched on and off with great rapidity. If a dog that had been leukophoresed for 6 hr and had restored its neutrophil count to normal was given a rest for 2 hr, the marrow stopped releasing neutrophils at a high rate, and a second series of leuko-phoreses could again depress the blood neutrophil count. An animal sub-jected to continuous leukophoresis over the same period would maintain its blood neutrophil count despite the losses. In these studies, no analysis of possible serum mediators of the effect was made, but it was suggested that the normal neutrophil secreted something that inhibited further release of neutrophils from bone marrow. Obviously, the results could be explained equally well by dogs' having a positive feedback control similar to that of Gordon's leukophoresed rats.

Some evidence that they do was obtained by Boggs and coworkers, who made dogs leukopenic by treating them with vinblastine, an alkaloid from the periwinkle that irreversibly damages mitosing cells.[9] Serum from these animals caused a rapid-onset, short-lived neutrophil leukocytosis in normal dogs, and serum from dogs treated with vinblastine either before or after the neutropenia was without effect. The authors went to some lengths to exclude endotoxin as an explanation; perhaps the most convincing of their experiments was to show that the effect was still obtained in dogs who had been rendered endotoxin-tolerant. It would be difficult to explain these results by the absence of an inhibitor, because presumably the normal recipient dog would have his own normal neutrophil level, and the normal level of any inhibitor they might produce.

During severe infections in man, the pool of mature neutrophils in the bone marrow may be completely depleted, so that the marrow shows essentially no forms more mature than the band cell. Under these circumstances, the blood neutrophil count falls from its elevated value to normal levels or below. Most of the neutrophils in the blood are band forms, and metamyelocytes and even myelocytes may be found. The cytoplasm of the cells may also show evidence of immaturity. "Toxic granules" are simply azurophil granules that have not been diluted out, as they are in normal development, and "Döhle bodies" are fragments of endoplasmic reticulum that a normal cell would have lost. These clinical observations are clear evidence that a hormone mobilizing mature neutrophils from the marrow is important in man; they would also suggest that during infection, cells are rushed through the myelocyte stage (because specific granule formation is defective). It was in patients such as these that Cronkite obtained his 48-hr myelocyte-to-blood times.

4.2.3. Chalones

A general problem in all metazoa is to understand how the growth of tissues is controlled so as to produce just the right amount of each, no more and no less. A skin wound leads to intense epithelial mitotic activity, which ceases at precisely the moment when the epidermis has been restored to its former level. If a lobe of the liver is removed, the other lobe grows until its weight is that of the normal liver, and then stops. Similar phenomena are seen after the removal of parts of endocrine organs, such as the thyroid, or mesodermal organs, such as the spleen; indeed, in the normal growth and development of each individual, some very precise control mechanisms must be responsible for the constancy of the normal anatomy and the relative weights of organs. Bullough and Lawrence, working with mouse skin, developed the concept that one controlling mechanism was a substance produced by normal epithelial cells in the prickle cell layer that inhibited mitosis in basal epithelial cells.[10] Thus, if a normal thickness of epidermis was present, the mitotic rate of the basal epidermal cells was low, but removal of the upper epidermis allowed basal cells to divide at an accelerated rate and to restore the deficiency.

The hypothetical substance was called a *chalone,* and substantial evidence for its existence was obtained: (1) Normal epidermis contains and secretes a substance that is not toxic for basal cells, but does inhibit DNA synthesis. (2) While much of its action is no doubt local, it does spread some distance in tissue, and may get into the bloodstream. (3) Epidermal chalone, like other chalones, is specific for its tissue of origin. When the skin is injured, only skin cells are stimulated to divide, not liver or blood cells.

All these features can be seen in the activities of the granulocytic chalone discovered by Rytomaa and his colleagues.[11] Chalone was obtained either directly from rat bone marrow cells or from the supernates of short-term neutrophil tissue cultures. It was purifed by ultrafiltration through a membrane that retained molecules of greater than 10,000 daltons, followed by gel filtration, paper electrophoresis, and thin-layer chromatography. The activity was tracked down to one of four small polypeptides, but it has not yet been possible to determine which is the crucial one, or its composition. Granulocytic chalone thus appears to be a single substance that is on the verge of being characterized biochemically.[12]

Early experiments were performed using rat bone marrow cultures *in vitro;* under these conditions, granulocyte precursors would take up tritiated thymidine for a few hours. Granulocytic chalone suppressed their thymidine uptake to about half normal, as assessed by autoradiography, while uptake by other bone marrow cells was unaffected. The specificity was confirmed by Paukovits, who separated bone marrow cells into different populations by centrifugation on Ficoll gradients and showed that only granulocyte precursors were inhibited.[12] The inhibition was found to be reversible, suggesting that this reaction was not a simple toxic one. Later experiments were done with cell populations in diffusion chambers in the mouse peritoneal cavity; chambers containing macrophages and lymphocytes took up thymidine normally, while granulocytes were inhibited. The most spectacular evidence for specificity was obtained in rats with the Shay chloroleukemia, which is a rapidly fatal malignant tumor of the granulocytic system. All rats treated with chalone showed evidence of regression of tumor, and some became apparently cured, with long-term survival and no evidence of tumor at autopsy. Of course, chalone by itself could not achieve this result; it would only stop the tumor from growing. But many tumors excite an immunological reaction that is known to be able to destroy relatively small numbers of cells, and it is conceivable that with tumor growth arrested, the immune system was responsible for the actual killing.[13]

The idea that granulocytic chalone has a physiological role was supported by experiments with serum from normal and leukophoresed rats. It was found that if normal serum was chromatographed on Sephadex G75, chalone activity was found in the effluent fractions corresponding to a molecular weight of 4000. In the region corresponding to a molecular weight of 30,000 was a protein that enhanced thymidine uptake by neutrophil precursors and was christened *antichalone*. Serum from leukophoresed rats showed much less chalone and more antichalone than the normal. Antichalone could not be extracted from neutrophils, and was presumed to arise from some other tissue.[11]

The mechanism of action of chalone appears to be an inhibition of the initiation of DNA synthesis; the main effect is to reduce the number of labeled cells, rather than the grain counts of those cells that are labeled. Cell death was not found; DNA synthesis returned to normal if the chalone was removed, and returned to normal spontaneously after 4 hr. Inhibition of uptake could be demonstrated also with [^{14}C]formate, [^{3}H]adenine, [^{35}SO$_4$]- or [^{14}C]aminoacids; this finding answers certain technical objections to the use of thymidine. The synthesis of RNA was also reduced.

The target cells for Rytomaa's chalone are the promyelocytes and myelocytes. There is a good deal of other evidence that important controls exist at this level. Thus, in a variety of acute infections in man, there is obvious hyperplasia of the myelocyte compartment, and if infection is chronic, the myeloid:erythroid ratio may rise from the normal 2:1 to 4 or 5:1. Not only are cell numbers increased, but also the mitotic indices. Most of the kinetic data reviewed in Chapter 3 is consistent with the view that the myelocyte compartment normally contains a substantial number of G_0 cells, and that these cells are a major source of extra neutrophils when the bone marrow is stimulated.

4.2.4. The Colony-Stimulating Factor

A control mechanism acting at the level of the cells committed to neutrophil production but not yet recognizable as neutrophil precursors is provided by the colony-stimulating factor (CSF). This factor has now been highly purified, though not to homogeneity. The best preparations to date suggest that it is a glycoprotein with a molecular weight of approximately 45,000, and that only 100 pg/ml is required to stimulate colony formation by bone marrow cells.[14]

Evidence for the physiological importance of CSF is indirect but substantial. The levels of CSF found in normal serum are about 10 times greater than those found to have significant stimulatory activity *in vitro*. Furthermore, CSF levels are higher than normal during various infections, and are unusually low in germ-free mice. Bacterial endotoxin and various other bacterial products cause rises in serum CSF, which may reach 100 times normal. After injections of endotoxin into mice, the number of hemopoietic stem cells in the bone marrow decreases, and the number of CFCs increases, suggesting that perhaps the stem cells have been stimulated to differentiate along the neutrophil pathway.

The main source for CSF in man appears to be lymphocytes and macrophages. Lymphocytes secrete CSF when stimulated by an antigen to which they are sensitized, or by general lymphocyte activators such as phytohemagglutinin. Endotoxin seems to be the best stimulus for macrophages. Since bacteria in general are good antigens, the potential for increased CSF production during infections is clearly present.

The gray collie dog has periodic swings in its blood neutrophil count, the values falling from normal or almost normal to very low over a period of a week or so, and then returning gradually to normal, when the cycle repeats. Periodic swings in urine CSF are observed, such that when the neutrophil count is high, the CSF level is low, and vice versa. It was suggested that the neutropenia triggered CSF production, which acted on the marrow to increase neutrophil supply after a lag due to the time required for production of mature cells. Once the neutrophil count was normal, CSF production shut off, and the decline began. A computer program was designed on the assumption that neutrophil production is controlled by a hormone that is produced in response to a low peripheral neutrophil count and acts on a precursor cell that cannot supply fresh neutrophils to the blood until many days have elapsed. The program predicted that cyclic variations in neutrophil count would occur with any mild bone marrow failure. Normal dogs were therefore treated with cyclophosphamide, and a dose was found that did not produce gross neutropenia, but cyclic variations similar to those seen in the spontaneous disease of the collie.[15]

There are substantial difficulties, however, in assuming that CSF is the only important substance regulating granulopoesis. Serum and urine levels are raised not only in bacterial infections, but also in viral infections, in which neutrophilia does not usually occur. In individual mice, there is very little correlation between serum levels of CSF and either CFC counts in bone marrow or peripheral neutrophil counts. Germ-free mice and mice treated with cortisone have very low levels of serum CSF, but neutrophil counts are not grossly abnormal. CSF levels are not raised in animals that have been rendered neutropenic by irradiation, even when neutrophil levels are steadily increasing. Last, although CSF injections do raise the neutrophil count of normal mice, the rise is well established at 24 hr and maximal at 48 hr, which is not really what one would expect for a stimulus acting on an early cell.

4.2.5. Stem Cell Controls

There must also be controls acting at the level of the multipotent stem cell. Most of these cells are not in cycle under normal conditions, but they can be stimulated to divide by any sudden demand for blood cells. A frequently used method is to shield one hind leg of a mouse and submit it to radiation that would otherwise be lethal. The mouse repopulates its bone marrow with cells from the shielded area, and during this process, the type of cell produced can be made to vary. Thus, if the mouse is transfused until its hematocrit is greater than 60%, more neutrophil precursors will be produced than otherwise.[16] The various differentiated pathways thus "compete for stem cells," and how they compete is unknown, although it is supposed that there may be a hormone, granulopoietin, that promotes differentiation along the granulocytic pathway. Certain tumors that cause neutrophil leukocytosis appear to do so by stimulating stem cells to divide, and it is suggested that the tumors may synthesize a hormone analogous to or identical with granulopoietin.

4.3. Summary

There is evidence for the existence of at least three factors that affect neutrophil delivery to the blood: One stimulates the mobilization of cells from the postmitotic pool in the marrow, chalone inhibits mitosis by recognizable neutrophil precursors, and CSF promotes mitosis by the committed precursor cells of neutrophil myeloblasts. None of these materials has been purified, and only biological assays are available. No coordinated attempt has been made to measure all three under the same circumstances, let alone under a wide range of experimental and clinical conditions. In consequence, it is not possible at present to give a complete description of how myelopoiesis is controlled, or even to be certain that any of the factors discussed above is physiologically important.

5

Inflammation and
Chemotaxis

We saw in Chapter 2 that neutrophils are mobile cells that spontaneously explore their environment in a random way and that can be induced to migrate in particular directions by suitable stimuli. This chapter will be concerned with the nature of the stimuli and with the processes by which neutrophils accumulate at inflammatory sites.

At a descriptive level, acute inflammation is thoroughly well understood, and every pathology textbook has a chapter on it. The essential early features are three: vasodilatation; increased vascular permeability; and sticking of leukocytes to the endothelium of small veins, with subsequent emigration of leukocytes into the tissues. Since many different agents of tissue damage cause very similar effects, it has long seemed likely that the noxious agent is merely a trigger that sets off a series of responses that are preprogrammed in the tissues. Because of this likelihood, an extensive search has been made in injured tissue for substances that cause vasodilatation, increased vascular permeability, or emigration of cells from the blood vessels. An embarrassingly large number of possible mediators has been found, all of which mimic one or another feature of the inflammatory response. It is difficult to show conclusively that any one of these substances is more important than the others, and the truth may be that all are involved to some extent. The type of evidence that one would like to have about a particular mediator of inflammation is that it is present in normal tissue in bound or in precursor form; that it is released in active form by noxious stimuli of several varieties; that the quantities found in inflamed tissue are adequate to explain one or more features of inflammation; that the time course of mediator release correlates with that of the feature in question; that the duration of action of the mediator is adequate to explain the duration of the feature; and, finally, that a specific antagonist of the putative mediator abolishes or diminishes part of the inflammatory response. Not many mediators can stand up to this searching kind of inquiry. It is also possible that some features of inflammation are due to the direct effect of injury on the vessels.

5.1. Inflammation

5.1.1. Gross Aspects

The classic macroscopic features of inflammation have been known for two thousand years: redness, heat, swelling, pain, and loss of function. The redness is due to dilatation of vessels, and has two components. In the injured area itself, small blood vessels are dilated, but they are also more permeable than usual. Plasma is lost into the tissue, red cell aggregates are left behind in the vessels, and flow is slower than normal and may even stop. The hemoglobin is thus partly deoxygenated, and the color is a dusky red. Around the injured area, there is arteriolar dilatation, with rapid flow of blood through normal vessels. This area is thus bright red (the "flare"). Thomas Lewis showed that the flare was an axon reflex and did not occur in an area where the sympathetic nerves had degenerated, while the vascular response in the injured area itself was independent of the nervous system.

Heat is a phenomenon that is probably confined to superficial inflamed sites. The normal temperature of hand skin is 30–32°C, and even the temperature of deep limb tissues such as muscle is 34–35°C during rest. When an athlete "warms up" before a race, he is really increasing the blood flow through his leg muscles and raising their temperature to a point at which they can function most effectively. Inflammation causes vasodilatation, and the temperature of the part approaches that of aortic blood. It thus seems hot by comparison with surrounding normal tissue.

Swelling is due to edema. The quantity of interstitial fluid in tissue is normally maintained by an equilibrium between the hydrostatic pressure in the small vessels and the osmotic pressure of the plasma proteins (Fig. 5.1). Blood plasma contains about 7 g protein/100 ml, whereas lymph, which is taken to represent the composition of interstitial fluid, frequently contains

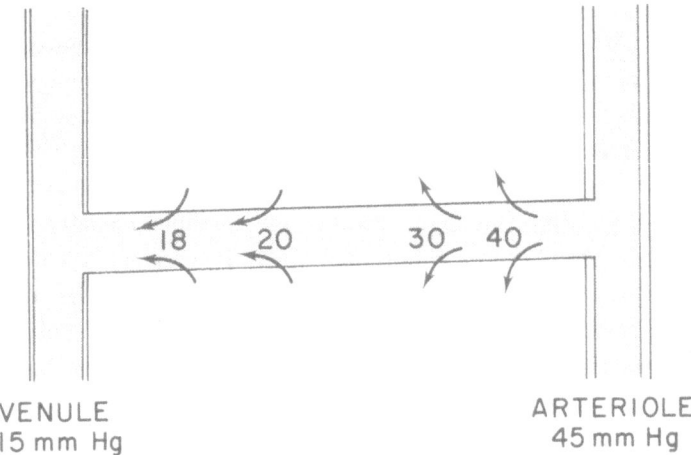

VENULE   ARTERIOLE
15 mm Hg   45 mm Hg

FIG. 5.1. The Starling equilibrium. This is a grossly simplified version of what actually goes on. Capillaries open and close; their cross-sectional area is not uniform; it is not clear that permeability is always the same; the pressure drop is probably not linear; there is a tissue pressure that tends to drive fluid into the capillaries, and a small osmotic pressure in tissue fluid that tends to draw fluid out. Nonetheless, it is a most important physiological concept, and is valid for large-scale work.

less than 0.5 g protein/100 ml. The difference in protein content is responsible for a net osmotic pressure of about 25 mm Hg, which tends to attract fluid from the tissues into the vessels. This osmotic pressure is opposed by the pressure in the vessels, which tends to filter off water and salts from the plasma into the tissues. At the arterial end of the capillaries, the pressure is 35–40 mm Hg, and there is a net filtration of water and salts outward into the tissue. At the venous end of the capillary, the pressure is lower, 15–20 mm Hg, so that the net movement of fluid is inward. In most resting tissues, this equilibrium is so evenly balanced that there is little or no accumulation of fluid in the tissue, and lymph flow is very small. Inflammation upsets this balance in two ways: Arterioles dilate, so that the hydrostatic pressure in vessels increases; capillaries become abnormally permeable, so that protein leaks into the interstitial fluid. Thus, the tissue becomes edematous, and the lymph draining from the area is proteinaceous and greatly increased in volume.

The cause of pain in inflamed areas is uncertain. Part of it is certainly due to increased tissue tension, especially once pus has formed. The macromolecules of dead cells break down into smaller fragments, which collectively have an increased osmotic pressure. Water is drawn in and the hydrostatic pressure may become very high, as anyone who has seen pus spurt when an abscess is incised can testify. But lesions such as burns, in which there is no pus, are often extremely painful, and it is thought that substances in inflamed tissue may directly stimulate nerve endings subserving pain sensation. Inflamed tissue has a high rate of glycolysis, so that lactic acid accumulates and the local pH falls. Dead and dying cells release intracellular electrolytes, principally potassium. Both K^+ and H^+ are painful when injected into the skin; whether the amounts available in injured tissue are adequate to cause pain is not known. Hyperosmolar solutions are painful immediately on injection, before disturbances of tissue tension could have arisen. Last, some of the inflammatory mediators cause pain in very low concentrations. Three such substances—serotonin, bradykinin, and prostaglandin E_1—will be discussed later.

5.1.2. Microscopic Aspects

Microscopic examination of living tissue during the development of the inflammatory response shows many subtleties not apparent in gross experiments. In the first place, Zweifach has shown that the capillaries are not merely identical tubes connecting arterioles and venules.[1] There are preferential channels for blood to flow between arteries and veins, and the true capillaries open off these channels. Each capillary has a short layer of muscle, the precapillary sphincter, at its origin, and during normal circumstances, most of these sphincters are closed. Every so often, a particular capillary will open up, and blood will flow through it for a time. This process is staggered for different capillaries, so that at any one time perhaps 5 or 10% of the total capillaries in resting tissue are open (Fig. 5.2). It is thought that the principal factors controlling flow through capillaries under normal circumstances are the local concentrations of oxygen and of tissue metabolites such as lactate and the hydrogen ion.

That the capillary bed when fully opened is enormously greater in cross-sectional area than either the arterioles or the venules is crucial in understanding a paradox of the inflammatory state. Overall, the blood flow through inflamed tissue is greatly increased, and yet the dominant microscopic feature is of vascular stasis, red cell sludging, and even total arrest of flow. What happens is that flow through the preferential channels is normal or increased, while the precapillary sphincters are paralyzed, all the capillaries are open, and flow in them is stagnant. In severely damaged tissue, even the through channels become occluded; here, one must suppose that the surrounding, less damaged tissue is carrying most of the blood flow.

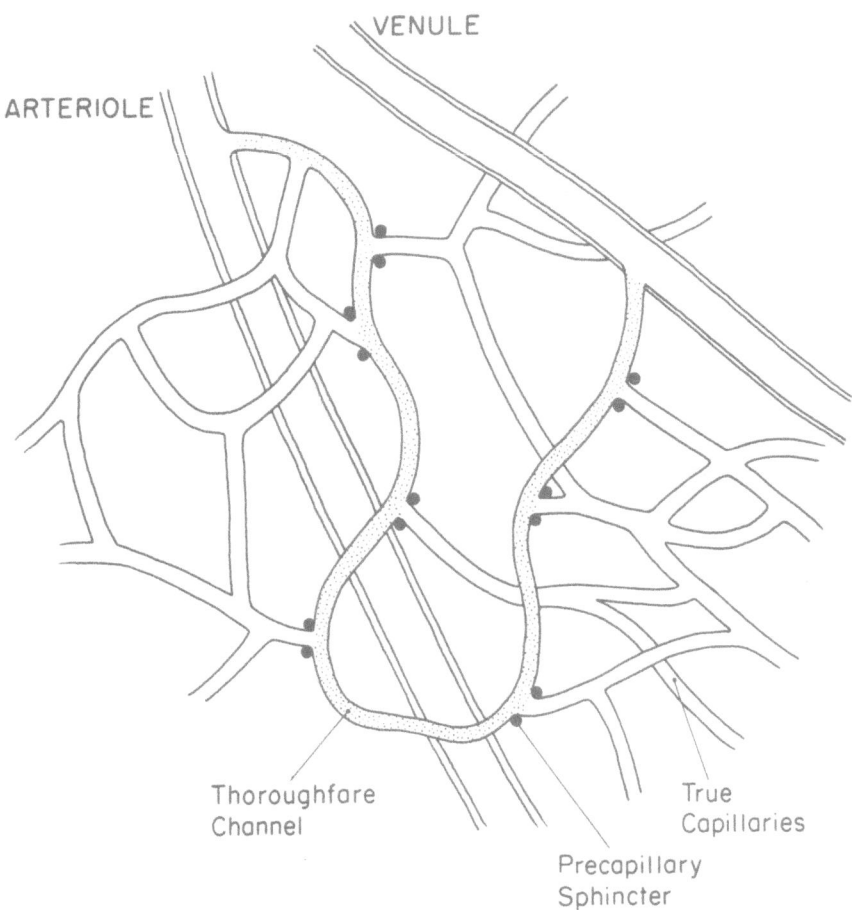

FIG. 5.2. The microcirculation: The preferential channel between artery and vein is dotted; the true capillaries open off it, and, at any one time, most of them are closed.

When the injury is sudden and distinct, such as a burn or mechanical stimulus, there is often a transient phase of arteriolar constriction. Injuries due to radiation and other gradual stimuli do not show this effect, and in any case it soon gives way to arteriolar dilatation, which may continue for hours. Many more capillaries are visible than in normal tissue. Within a few minutes of injury, the smallest venules show a highly significant change. Under normal circumstances, neutrophils and other leukocytes tend to travel in the periphery of the bloodstream, while red cells travel in the faster, central portion. Since the leukocytes travel peripherally, they naturally bump against the endothelium from time to time, and even in tissue that is kept in a state as close to physiological as possible, neutrophils stick to the endothelium momentarily. The motion is a rolling one, in which the cell moves slowly over the endothelium, presumably driven by the force of the bloodstream, and is normally concluded when the cell detaches from the endothelium and rejoins the circulation. Early in inflammation, the adhesion of leukocytes to venule walls increases, the cells roll more slowly and take longer to detach, and the venule wall becomes progressively pavemented with white blood cells.[2] Soon, the cells no longer detach, but wander about on the endothelium; shortly after that, they begin to penetrate the venule walls, and pass into the tissue.

The adhesion of white cells to venule walls produces substantial obstruction to blood flow, and pressures in the capillaries rise to arteriolar levels, as has been confirmed by direct measurement.[3] This increased pressure in itself promotes loss of fluid into the tissues, and, in addition, the damaged capillary walls are unable to retain plasma proteins. Masses of red cells are left in the vessels, and since the viscosity of blood rises rapidly with the hematocrit, flow slows even more. Sometimes capillaries actually burst, and small hemorrhages result.

5.1.3. Increased Vascular Permeability

From the earliest stage of inflammation, increased permeability of small blood vessels is demonstrable. The usual means of measuring this increase is to label a plasma protein, commonly albumin, with some substance that is easily measured. This substance may be a dye, which can be seen or measured spectrophotometrically, a radioactive isotope, or any other convenient substance. The linkage to protein need not be covalent as long as the association constant is high. Since normal capillaries do not allow much protein to enter tissue, the dye or radioactivity will accumulate only in inflamed areas, and, within limits, the amount of accumulation is proportional to the degree of the insult. For example, it is possible to find a dose range in which the amount of Evans blue dye that enters a skin site varies directly as the logarithm of the amount of histamine injected. A second method is to inject into the bloodstream some foreign substance, the size of which is such that it is normally retained within vessels. Substances used have ranged from colloidal carbon and mercuric sulfide particles, which may reach 0.1 μm in diameter, down to enzymes such as horseradish peroxidase, which has a molecular weight of about 40,000 daltons. Opaque substances are viewed directly by light or electron microscopy; enzymes are detected histochemically.

Capillary permeability is a complex subject, and those interested in the details can find them in several excellent reviews.[4] Basically, the capillary wall is composed of flattened endothelial cells. The cell membrane is of the usual mammalian type, and adjacent cells are separated by a cleft about 250 Å wide. In some areas, there are tight junctions, where the gap between cells narrows to about 100 Å. The endothelial cells have an external, probably glycoprotein, coat that also fills the clefts. In some capillaries, the endothelial cells are fenestrated, and in these areas, the glycoprotein external layer bridges the gap to form a "diaphragm." The cytoplasm of endothelial cells contains many vesicles. Most of these vesicles are wholly intracytoplasmic, but some open onto either the luminal or the external surface as pits called *caveolae*. It has been suggested that diaphragms are produced when a vesicle opens onto both surfaces simultaneously. Outside the endothelium is a basement membrane, and outside that again is a discontinuous layer of cells with branching processes called *pericytes* (Fig. 5.3).

Normally, the major barrier to the diffusion of macromolecules from capillaries appears to be the glycoprotein material that fills the fenestrations and the intercellular clefts. Most fluid exchange occurs through the clefts. Quite large particles may be enfolded in cytoplasmic vesicles, transported across the cell, and released to the exterior when the vesicle fuses with the outer cell membrane. However, most investigators do not believe that this route is a major one for egress of substances from blood vessels. The basement membrane seems to be more porous than the glycoprotein layer and probably does not hold up water, small molecules, and what protein manages to get through the primary barrier. However, if large particles or cells do exit from injured capillaries, they may be retained around the capillary but inside the basement membrane as a kind of sleeve.

There is now a consensus that the primary lesion in inflammation is a separation of the endothelial cells, and that both protein and cells leave the vessels through the junctions. Majno points out that most substances that increase the permeability of small vessels are also capable of stimulating smooth muscle to contract.[5] He believes that endothelial cells may contain actomyosin filaments, and that they may contract actively after injury. However this may be, Majno and Palade showed the site of emigration of colloidal carbon from blood vessels by injecting a rat with carbon intrave-

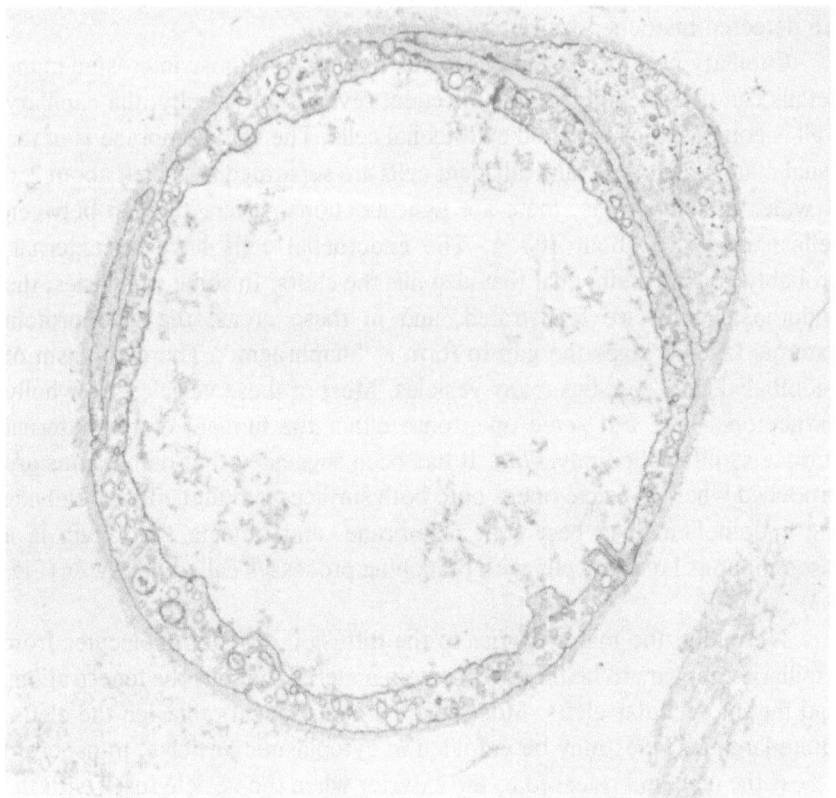

FIG. 5.3. A capillary from mouse diaphragm (electron micrograph, ×17,100). Two endothelial cells with junctions are seen. The cells contain numerous vesicles, and caveolae can be seen. The basement membrane and pericyte are also shown. (From Luft, J. H. *The Inflammatory Process*, Vol. 2, Academic Press, New York, 1973, Chap. 2.[4])

nously, and injecting an inflammatory mediator into the cremaster muscle. After a suitable time, usually about an hour, the muscle was excised, cleared, and examined by light microscopy. Throughout the preparations, small venules were outlined with carbon, and detailed examination showed that the particles filled the intercellular clefts, but had been unable to pass the basement membrane, and had therefore moved sideways over the external surface of the endothelial cells to form a more or less complete investing coat. Dye-labeled protein left by the same route, but penetrated the basement membrane and passed out into the tissues. At no time was it possible to see more vesicles or bigger vesicles, so there was no evidence that vesicular transport accounted for more than a tiny fraction of the leakage.[6] These results have been confirmed in several laboratories.

In most types of injuries, there is a more or less clear separation of increased permeability into two phases.[7] The first comes on almost immediately after injury, affects mainly the smallest venules, and lasts only about 30 min. Beginning at about an hour after injury, there is a second phase of increased permeability that often lasts for hours or days. There is much variation in detail in these phases: In severe injury, they are telescoped together; in continuing injuries such as bacterial infections or the response to ultraviolet radiation, the later phase is exaggerated and prolonged. For the present purposes, it will suffice to say that the later phase appears to affect the true capillaries instead of, or as well as, the venules. The fundamental lesion is the same: separation of endothelial cells and emigration of plasma and particles between them.

5.1.4. Emigration of Cells from Vessels

Neutrophils and monocytes also leave the vessels through gaps between endothelial cells. By light microscopy, marginated cells can be observed to move about on the vessel wall, presumably searching for a suitable site for egress. Neither the gap nor the pseudopod that the cell puts through it can be seen by light microscopy, but beautiful electron micrographs from Florey's laboratory show that in all cases, if serial sections are studied, the pseudopod passes between contiguous endothelial cells, and that the cell membranes of the endothelial cells and of the neutrophil remain separate and distinct[8] (Fig. 5.4). Once through the endothelial layer, the cell may penetrate the basement membrane directly, but commonly it passes sideways for some distance in the subendothelial plane, and sometimes a number of neutrophils can be seen temporarily trapped in this site. By light microscopy, it can be seen that several neutrophils may exit from the same site, and less often a red cell or two may follow, presumably expelled passively by the blood pressure.

The mechanism of neutrophil exit is not known. The gaps are never very large, 0.1–0.4 μm wide, through of course their length is indefinite. Observation of the actively amoeboid movement of living cells suggests that considerable energy is required to force a 10-μm cell through such a small opening. If the motion is analogous to that on glass, one would expect that the pseudopod would flow out more or less passively and subsequently

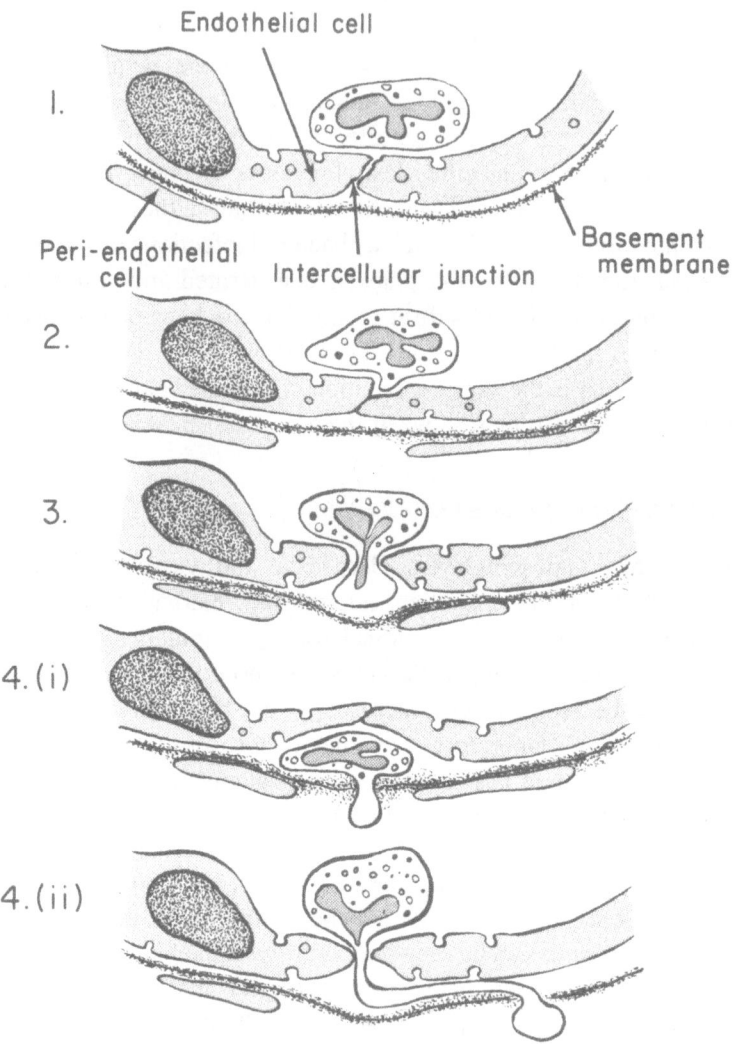

FIG. 5.4. The mechanism of neutrophil exit from venules. The pseudopod sometimes passes more or less straight out of the vessel, as illustrated in 4.(i). Sometimes, as in 4.(ii), it runs along the wall of the vessel for a considerable distance before making its exit through the basement membrane. [The original electron micrographs can be seen in Marchesi, V. T., and Florey, H. W., *Q. J. Exp. Physiol.* **45**:343 (1960),[5] and Marchesi, V. T., *Q. J. Exp. Physiol.* **46**:115 (1961).]

pull the rest of the cell through. Alternatively, the cell might contract filaments on its luminal side and force the pseudopod out hydraulically. Data to resolve the point are not available, but it is certain that emigration is an active process, because it has been observed in inflamed areas in which the arterial supply has been cut off, or even when the animal itself is dead. Whether the cell has any enzymes that degrade either the glycoprotein matrix filling the intercellular junctions or the basement membrane is uncertain; if so, they do not leave obvious defects in either.

We do not know why neutrophils stick to inflamed endothelium. The change is one in the tissue, and the circulating cells themselves are entirely normal. That they are has always seemed likely, because it was inconceivable that the blood cells exposed to the original injury could possibly return to the inflamed site after being diluted in the whole circulating volume. It has now been formally proved by Grant and Epstein, who found a normal inflammatory response in tissue perfused with a saline solution, the blood being readmitted only when the injury was completed.[9] It is uncertain whether the endothelium can be damaged directly or whether it merely responds to chemical mediators that develop in the tissue and diffuse into the vessel. Attempts are now being made to persuade endothelium to grow as a monolayer in tissue culture; if these attempts are successful, a direct attack on many problems will be possible. There is no obvious ultrastructural abnormality about the luminal surface of inflamed endothelial cells in most locations, although in special areas such as the pancreas, the development of processes projecting into the lumen and apparently trapping passing cells has been claimed.[10] Florey described the momentary arrest of red cells on invisible intravascular spikes in inflamed vessels of rabbit ear chambers, so there may be something in this idea.[11] It seems clear that palisading and emigration of neutrophils are not connected with increased vascular permeability in any obligatory way; minimal inflammatory stimuli may cause leukocyte sticking without measurable increase in permeability; in more severe inflammations, the time course of leukocyte emigration is not necessarily correlated to either phase of increased permeability; and, finally, some substances can induce leukocyte sticking without change in permeability, and vice versa. It is less clear whether palisading and emigration of neutrophils are different reactions or merely different degrees of response to the same stimuli. It is certainly possible to produce palisading alone by minimal injury or by low concentrations of certain inflammatory mediators. All these latter substances are chemotactic for neutrophils when tested *in vitro*. If palisading and emigration are in fact the same response, one is then in the slightly awkward position of assuming that one and the same substance acts on endothelial cells to promote contraction and the creation of gaps, and acts on neutrophils to direct them to move in a particular direction. It would be neater to suppose that one substance mediates sticking of cells to vessel walls, and that chemotactic agents draw them out once they have palisaded.

5.1.5. Mediators of Inflammation

We have several times mentioned the inflammatory mediators, but have so far skirted the problem of just what they are. They can be divided into substances that promote increased vascular permeability and substances that promote leukocyte emigration. Since the permeability factors are only tangentially relevant to the neutrophil, they will be reviewed very briefly.

(a) Histamine and Serotonin. It seems likely that the cause of the early increase in permeability is histamine or, in some species, serotonin (Fig. 5.5). Histamine is produced by the decarboxylation of histidine, a one-step reaction. Serotonin is derived from tryptophan by a two-step reaction: hydroxylation at the 5 position, followed by decarboxylation of the side chain.

Histamine is available in all tissues, stored in the granules of mast cells. It is also found in the granules of basophil leukocytes and in platelets; certain immunological reactions such as systemic anaphylaxis and immune complex diseases appear to involve blood histamine, rather than tissue histamine. A large number of noxious stimuli and an even larger number of substances will cause mast cells to degranulate and liberate histamine into tissue. In most species, including the guinea pig, the rabbit, and man, less than 1 μg of histamine produces increased vascular permeability that comes on within a minute or two and lasts for 15–20 min. Histamine has been isolated from experimental pleural effusions in amounts and at times adequate to explain the early fluid accumulation.[12] The compound 48/80 causes mast cells to degranulate; after injection of this material, the earliest phase of inflammation is suppressed. Antihistamine drugs such as mepyramine that block the action of histamine also suppress the early phase of various experimental inflammations.

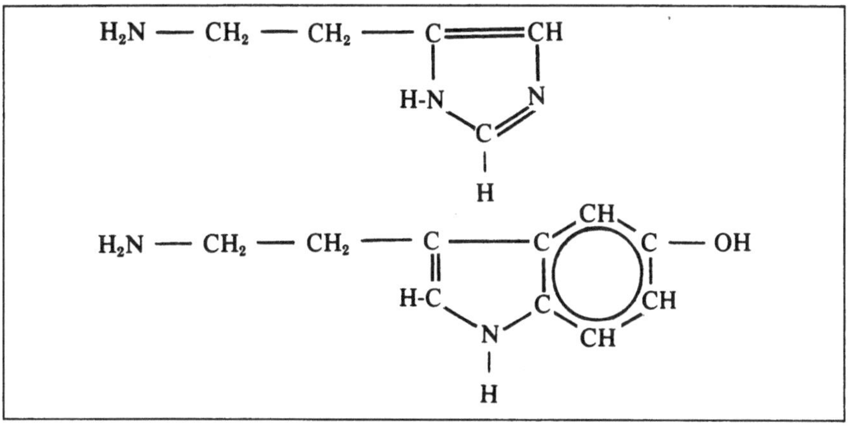

FIG. 5.5. Histamine (above) and serotonin.

Serotonin is also found in the granules of mast cells, platelets, and basophils, and is released by the same stimuli. In species that are not very sensitive to histamine, such as the rat, serotonin appears to be the main cause of the early phase; the type of evidence is similar to that for histamine.

Histamine cannot be responsible for long-continued vascular permeability, even if one were to assume that it is released continuously in inflammatory sites. The response to repeated injections shows tachyphylaxis, or a progressive decline in the response to the same dose until eventually no response occurs to almost any dose. Furthermore, there is evidence from pleural effusions caused by turpentine that histamine release is no longer demonstrable after 30 min, and 48/80 and antihistamines have no effect on the delayed permeability response.[12] Similar evidence suggests that serotonin can be important only early on.

(b) The Kinins. Another group of substances causing increased vascular permeability in submicrogram doses is the kinins. A simple experiment that dramatically demonstrates most of the features of this system is to aspirate 5 or 10 ml of blood from a man's brachial artery into a glass syringe and reinject it immediately. The exposure to glass lasts less than 10 sec, but it causes an intense vasodilatation in the forearm and hand that comes on at once and lasts for several minutes. The system of reactions that produces this effect has now been worked out in fair detail (Fig. 5.6). Normal serum contains a protein—the Hageman factor, or Factor XII—that undergoes a

cleavage when exposed to glass and certain materials of more biological interest, such as collagen, vascular basement membrane, and bacteria.[13] One of the products is an anionic protein, molecular weight 32,000 daltons, that converts another plasma protein, prekallikrein, to the active enzyme kallikrein. Kallikrein acts on a third plasma protein, kininogen, splitting off bradykinin. The system is autocatalytic, in that kallikrein is a powerful activator of the Hageman factor. How the initial reaction occurs is uncertain. It may be that Hageman factor on glass exposes an active site that activates prekallikrein, and that cleavage of the Hageman factor molecule is associated only with the amplification step.

Bradykinin is a nonapeptide; its sequence is known and it has been synthesized (Fig. 5.7). It is the most potent inflammatory agent known in most species, causing increased vascular permeability in doses of less that 0.1 μg. Kallikreins are found in many tissues and also in urine; they act on kininogen to form lysylbradykinin, the potency and activity of which are similar to those of bradykinin. Other proteolytic enzymes such as trypsin and plasmin cause the release of bradykinin from kininogen. In the past, several different kininogens of differing molecular weights have been reported, but it now looks as though these may have been polymers of a single glycoprotein.[14]

The kinin system is ubiquitous and easily activated, and does not show tachyphylaxis. Bradykinin has been demonstrated in burned skin. Nonetheless, it has been impossible to provide unequivocal evidence that kinin generation is crucial to either phase of increased permeability. In particular, human families exist who are deficient in either the Hageman factor or in prekallikrein (the "Fletcher factor"). Plasma from these patients is unable to generate kinins, but they do not suffer from any obvious susceptibility to infectious illnesses.

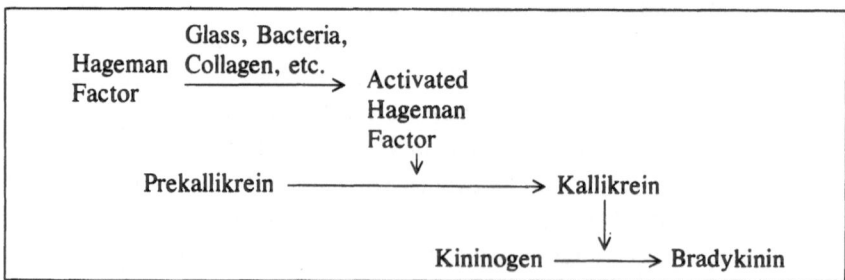

FIG. 5.6. Kinin generation in plasma. Plasma kallikrein splits off the nonapeptide bradykinin from kininogen. Tissue kallikreins have different specificities, and most commonly yield lysylbradykinin.

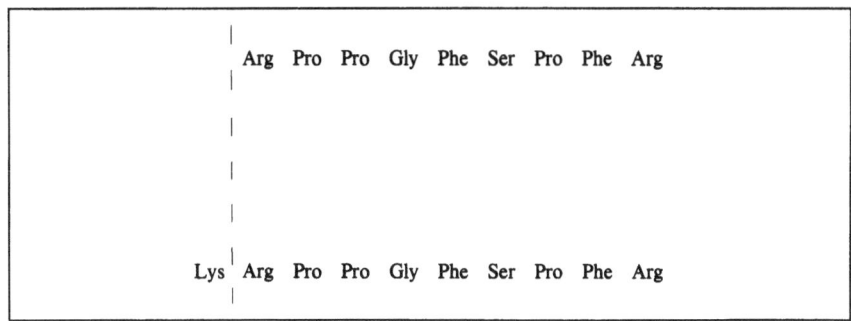

FIG. 5.7. Structures of bradykinin and lysylbradykinin. Other kinins certainly exist, and presumably result from splitting of the kininogen chain at other points.

There is some evidence that kinins are responsible for the early portion of the delayed permeability response, about 1–2 hr after injury. Animals depleted of histamine, serotonin, and kinins do not develop edema until nearly 3 hr after mild burning, whereas normally the delayed response is under way at 1 hr.[15] However, the intensity and duration of the delayed phase as a whole are hardly altered.

(c) Prostaglandins. The latest candidates for the role of mediator of the main, delayed, increase in vascular permeability are the prostaglandins. These are a family of acidic lipids that are synthesized in inflammatory tissue from fatty acid precursors. At least 19 prostaglandins are known at present, several of which produce leakage of carbon and other colloidal particles in doses of less than 1 μg. Prostaglandin E_1 also causes pain, which may last for hours after subcutaneous injection. The strongest evidence that prostaglandins are important inflammatory mediators has come from the work of Vane, who showed that aspirin, phenylbutazone, indomethacin, and similar antiinflammatory drugs had a powerful inhibitory effect on prostaglandin synthesis by various tissue homogenates.[16] These drugs do not affect the early phase of increased permeability, but do suppress the delayed phase. Examination of experimental inflammations caused by turpentine and carrageenan showed that prostaglandins appeared in the edema fluid after 30 min, and that the concentration built up until it reached a maximum at about 16 hr. The concentrations were entirely adequate to explain the observed increased permeability. The relative antiinflammatory potencies of drugs in these experimental inflammations correlate quite closely with their inhibitory actions on prostaglandin synthesis.

The permeability induced by prostaglandins resembles that due to histamine, serotonin, and the kinins in that the principal vessels affected are the small venules. Hurley has suggested that increased permeability of the true capillaries is due to the direct effect of injury on them, and that no chemical mediator is involved.[17] Whether this view is correct is not yet clear. Nor is it clear which cells synthesize prostaglandins in inflamed tissue. Willoughby and his colleagues found that during carrageenan edema, prostaglandins were indeed released, and seemed to be causally related to the increased permeability. However, if either neutrophils or monocytes were prevented from emigrating into the tissue, the delayed phase was diminished; if neither type of cell could emigrate, edema did not develop.[18] Since both neutrophils and monocytes are known to synthesize prostaglandins, this finding suggested that the prostaglandins important in this variety of inflammation were synthesized by the invading cells. Other workers using other systems have found perfectly normal inflammatory responses in the total absence of neutrophils, so the point is unresolved at present. However, all tissues investigated so far have proved to possess the capacity for prostaglandin synthesis, so one would not imagine *a priori* that neutrophils were always essential.

5.2. Chemotaxis

Of the mediators discussed so far, only prostaglandins (especially PGE_1) cause emigration of neutrophils into skin.[19] Actually, this emigration is a very bad way to test the chemotactic effect of any substance, because the small vessels are so delicate that even the injection of substances that ought to be innocuous, such as normal saline, leads to some emigration of neutrophils. Furthermore, there are two apparently insurmountable objections to observing the response to intradermal or subcutaneous injections: First, it is entirely possible that a substance that attracts neutrophils into the skin does so indirectly, by stimulating tissue cells to manufacture some endogenous mediator. Second, even if a substance acts directly, it by no means follows that leukocytes accumulate in the skin because they are attracted by the substance. If one hangs a flypaper in the center of a room full of flies, one soon discovers that most of the flies are on the paper. The reason is not that they are attracted to the paper, but that once they alight on it, they find it impossible to leave. That this is not merely an idle thought was demonstrated by Allison, Smith, and Wood, who studied the response to microburns in the rabbit ear chamber.[20] A platinum wire passed through the center of the chamber could be heated by touching it with a soldering iron. The resulting injury caused an inflammatory response, and it was observed that neutrophils would even preferentially emigrate from the side of the vessel nearest the burn. However, once in the tissue, they had no tendency to migrate in any particular direction. After many hours, they did accumulate around the wire, presumably because, once there, they became immobilized.

Most of what we know about chemotactic substances has been learned by the use of *in-vitro* techniques, and the evidence that the agents that are chemotactic *in vitro* are actually important *in vivo* is spotty. Furthermore, experiments *in vitro* are fraught with all kinds of pitfalls, and it is terribly easy to get misleading results. For example, everyone agrees that bacteria are chemotactic, and yet rarely does one find that substances alleged to attract neutrophils have been cultured and are sterile. Nor is sterility alone adequate, because bacterial products, such as endotoxin, may persist in the solutions even though the bacteria that synthesized them have been removed. Then, the techniques themselves leave much to be desired; their very multiplicity means that no one of them can be satisfactory. Almost all are difficult to quantitate, and it is impossible to obtain the same numerical values from tests on different batches of cells. In fact, although chemotaxis of neutrophils was described in the nineteenth century, it was not until 1953 that Henry Harris demonstrated to everyone's satisfaction that it was a genuine phenomenon.[21]

5.2.1. Chemotaxis on Glass Slides

Harris reviewed and dismissed all previous attempts to demonstrate chemotaxis *in vitro,* and introduced a new technique. Neutrophils were layered onto glass slides in autologous serum, and photographs were taken through a dark-field microscope at regular intervals, the exposures all being superimposed on one negative. Each cell produced an appearance reminiscent of a snail track as it moved about, while the background remained dark. In the absence of bacteria, the snail tracks had a random distribution, but in the presence of a clump of bacteria, all the tracks converged directly on the organisms (Fig. 5.8). The only effective stimuli found by Harris were bacteria; all bacteria tested attracted neutrophils, even those such as the tubercle bacillus that characteristically cause a mononuclear type of inflammatory response. Pieces of sterile muscle, liver, kidney, and various other body tissues including neutrophils were ignored. That normal tissues and tissue extracts did not attract neutrophils was the key to understanding

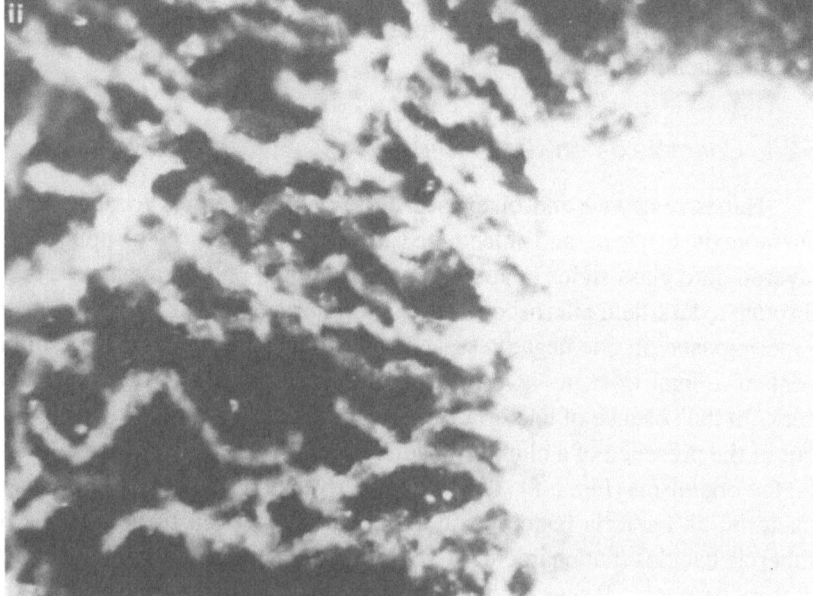

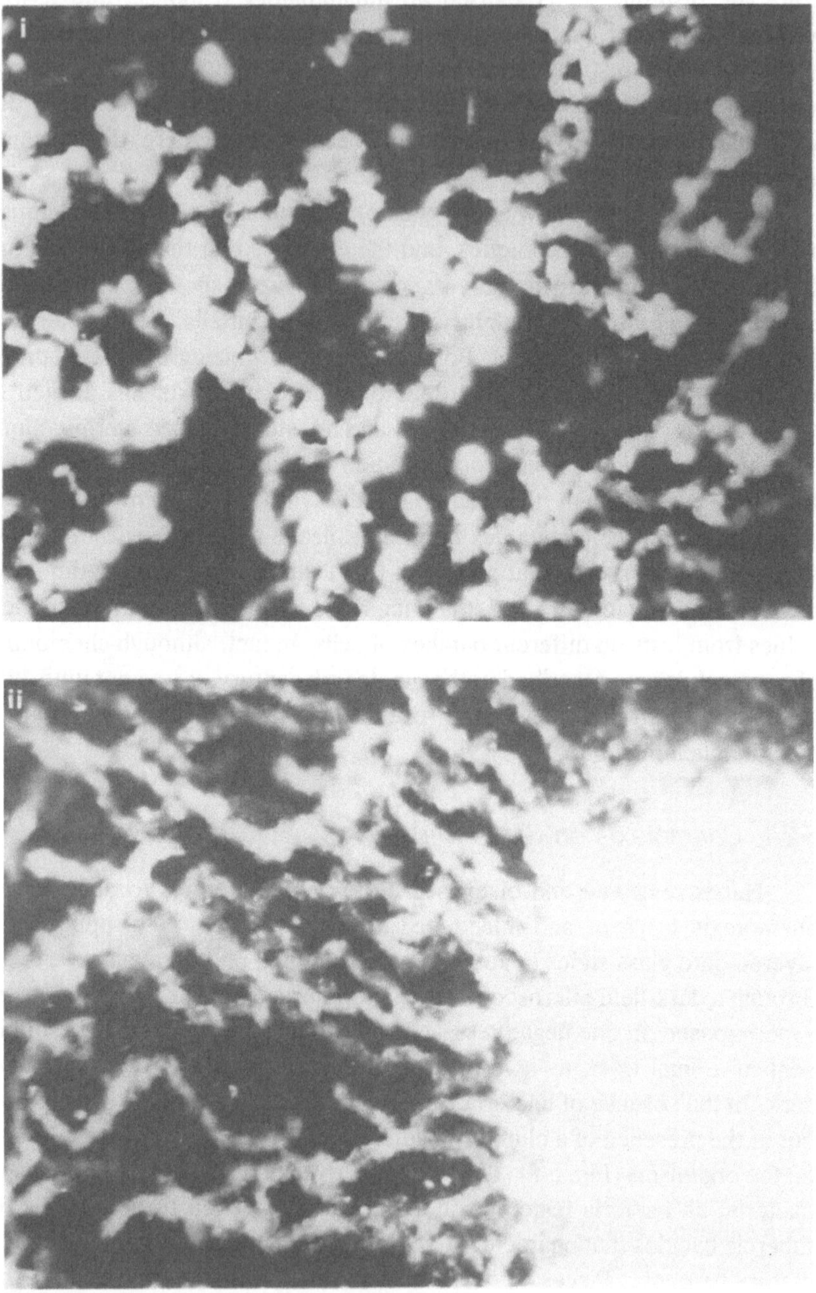

FIG. 5.8. Chemotaxis on glass slides. In (i), neutrophils are wandering at random; in (ii), a clump of *Staphylococcus albus* is to the right, and all the cells are converging on it. [From Harris, H., *J. Pathol. Bacteriol.* **66:**135 (1953).]

Allison's results in the rabbit ear chamber. Neutrophils emigrated from the vessels because the vessels were damaged, but once in the tissues, there was no reason they should migrate in any particular direction.

The conclusion that tissue components are not chemotactic was challenged by Ryan and Hurley, who showed that severely burned tissue was chemotactic when examined by the Harris technique, but that the range over which attraction would occur was only about 100 μm.[22] Bacteria would attract over distances of 500–700 μm. They also showed that normal tissue incubated in serum for 3–4 hr became chemotactic, though tissue incubated in saline was not. Thus, tissue can be chemotactic under at least two circumstances: (1) when the injury is severe enough to actually kill cells, and (2) when dead tissue interacts with serum.

Harris's technique was exacting and not easily quantitated, and besides, it was ill adapted to determining what substances mediated the observed phenomenon.

5.2.2. The Boyden Chamber

A major step forward was made by Boyden, who devised the first apparatus in which it was possible to test soluble substances for chemotactic activity.[23] He used a chamber that consisted of an upper and a lower half separated by a membrane (Fig. 5.9). The lower compartment was completely filled with the solution that was to be tested for activity, and a suspension of neutrophils was then layered onto the upper surface. The chambers were sealed and incubated at 37°C.

Preliminary experiments were done with tuberculin, which is a protein purified from culture filtrates of the tubercle bacillus. Few or no neutrophils crossed the membrane when saline was used in the lower chamber, but many crossed when tuberculin was added. This crossing might have represented a mere stimulation of motility; this possibility was excluded by putting the tuberculin in both upper and lower compartments. When there was no gradient of tuberculin concentration, the cells did not cross the membrane. In all these experiments, semiquantitative results could be obtained by staining the cells with Ehrlich's hematoxylin, clearing the membranes in xylene, and counting the number of cells that had completely traversed the membrane in 10 random fields.

Boyden was interested in finding out whether or not antigen–antibody complexes were chemotactic. He found that if a mixture of human serum albumin and specific antiserum was placed in the lower compartment, large numbers of neutrophils crossed the filter. If antiserum to human serum

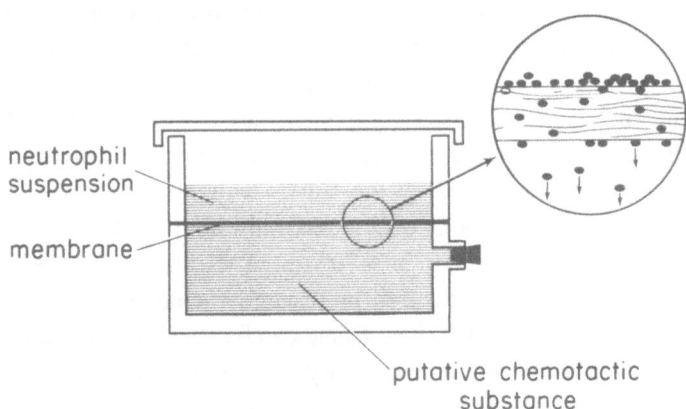

FIG. 5.9. The Boyden chamber (1962).

albumin was mixed with egg albumin, no migration was seen. Similarly, antibody to ovalbumin attracted neutrophils when it was mixed with ovalbumin, but not when mixed with human serum albumin. It was further found that if the amount of antigen was varied while the antibody was held constant, chemotaxis was strongest when the complexes were in the equivalence zone. If precipitation was allowed to go to completion, the clear supernate was chemotactic, whereas washed complexes were not. If the serum was heated at 56°C for 30 min, precipitation of antigen was unimpaired, but chemotactic activity failed to develop. However, once soluble chemotactic activity had developed, that activity was heat-stable.

These results showed that during the course of specific antigen–antibody reactions, some heat-labile component of serum was activated and gave rise to a soluble, heat-stable chemotactic factor. Since complement is heat-labile, and is most efficiently fixed by complexes in the equivalence zone, Boyden suggested that perhaps complement was involved.

Boyden's technique has undergone innumerable modifications in detail, and almost every investigator has used his own variant. The major disadvantage of the original method was the necessity of counting the cells that had crossed the membrane, which was difficult, tedious, and time-consuming. Furthermore, the agreement between replicate chambers was far from perfect. It turned out that at least some of the variation was due to the fact that some cells that had crossed the membrane relinquished their hold, fell into the fluid filling the lower chamber, and were not counted. Last, there is a substantial motility factor in these assays. Even in the absence of any chemotactic gradient, neutrophils will eventually cross the membrane, and any substance that stimulates their random motility may therefore speed up this process and appear to be chemotactic. Few investigators are as meticulous about their controls as Boyden was, and much sloppy work has been published.

A modified Boyden procedure that goes some distance toward meeting these objections has recently been described by Gallin and his co-workers.[24] They used two filters, and counted only neutrophils that migrated right through the upper filter and onto the lower one. They also labelled the neutrophils with ^{51}Cr, so that the degree of migration could be quantitated by gamma counting. Keller also uses two filters, but thinks that accurate results are obtainable only by counting both the cells on the lower surface of the upper filter and the cells on the second filter.[25] Naturally, this cannot be done by using labeled cells, so the technique is even more laborious than the original.

5.2.3. The System of Zigmond and Hirsch

Another approach to the problem of measuring chemotaxis with membranes is that of Zigmond and Hirsch.[26] When leukocytes are layered on top of a filter, it is to be expected that some of them will migrate into it in a purely random manner. Since these cells are not moving in any directed way, they will change direction from time to time. The motion can therefore be described by the same random walk theory that fits their two-dimensional movement on the surface of glass slides. In fact, the equations used to describe the diffusion of a protein or other macromolecule from a front such as that created in the Tiselius electrophoresis apparatus give a very adequate fit to the experimental data for neutrophil migration through membranes. It turned out that the easiest and most reproducible parameter to measure was the mean distance from the top of the filter to the furthest point within the filter where it was possible to see at least two cells in focus. The experiments were always concluded at a time when the cell front was still well within the substance of the filter.

The observations were now repeated, using various concentrations of a putative chemotactic factor. This particular one was the supernate from neutrophils that had been allowed to phagocytose antigen–antibody complexes. It was not further characterized, except that it was heat-stable and nondialyzable.

Zigmond and Hirsch set up various concentrations of their factor, both

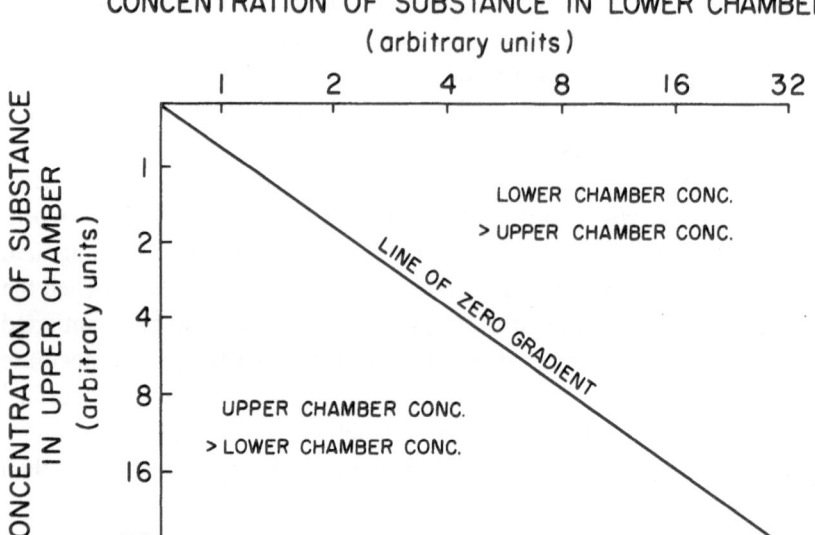

FIG. 5.10. The membrane system of Zigmond and Hirsch. The values plotted in the table are distances to the cell front after a fixed time interval.

above and below the membrane, and tabulated the results in the fashion indicated (Fig. 5.10). At the top left corner is the control value with no factor in either chamber. Along the diagonal is a series of motility figures with increasing concentrations of factor, but without a concentration gradient; these values allow one to assess the effect of the factor on motility alone. The factor they were using definitely stimulated motility in low concentrations, but inhibited it as the concentration rose. Above and to the right of the diagonal was an area in which the concentration of factor in the lower chamber exceeded that in the upper. Cells in these conditions moved faster than diffusion theory would have suggested, indicating that positive chemotaxis had occurred. Below and to the left of the diagonal was an area in which the concentration in the upper chamber exceeded that in the lower. Motility values in this area were low, suggesting that the cells had been held back by the attractive stimulus above. This type of analysis seems to be the most comprehensive yet available for analyzing the response of neutrophils to chemical agents.

5.2.4. Chemotactic Substances

The techniques of measuring chemotaxis may be defective and subject to error, but certain substances have been found to be chemotactic for neutrophils by many different groups of workers, and for some of them, there is evidence that this activity is important in living animals. They include complement components, immunoglobulin fragments, fragments of fibrinogen and collagen, kallikrein, and prostaglandin E_1. All bacteria produce chemotactic substances; some require the presence of serum for activity, others do not. Many proteolytic enzymes generate chemotactic activity if allowed access to serum; among these are the enzymes of neutrophil lysosomes, and it seems probable that this is of physiological importance. A number of mechanisms tending to damp down chemotaxis have also been discovered.

(a) Bacteria. Everyone who has attempted to demonstrate chemotaxis by any technique has found that bacteria were chemotactic for neutrophils. Why this is so is a little difficult to explain, given that the structure of bacterial surfaces is so varied. The possibilities appear to be five in number: (i) Bacteria produce soluble substances which act directly on neutrophils to induce chemotaxis. (ii) Soluble factors are produced which interact with complement components to generate chemotactic activity. (iii) Bacterial bodies react with serum components and generate chemotactic factors. (iv) Neutrophils encountering bacteria by chance liberate substances which summon other neutrophils to the scene. (v) Neutrophils meeting bacteria by chance liberate substances which act on serum components to generate chemotactic factors. There is some evidence for all of these possibilities:

(i) Directly Acting Soluble Components. Keller and Sorkin showed that both *Escherichia coli* and *Staphylococcus aureus* liberate into the culture medium small molecules, apparently protein in nature, with molecular weights in the 3000–4000 dalton range.[27] The tuberculin used by Boyden and already discussed is of the same general type. These substances are not likely to be or to be contaminated with bacterial endotoxin; endotoxin as usually obtained has a molecular weight of $>1,000,000$ daltons and its essential component is a glycolipid; endotoxin is chemotactic only in the presence of serum, whereas these small proteins are directly chemotactic; endotoxin is not a component of either *S. aureus* or *Mycobacterium tuberculosis*. It seems very unlikely that widely disparate bacteria would produce identical small proteins with the function of summoning cells to encompass their destruction, and indeed evidence was obtained that these substances are *not* identical. One therefore has the opposite problem of how the neutrophil recognizes and reacts to completely different stimuli. Two possible explanations are to be found in the work of Wilkinson and of Becker, which is discussed below.

(ii) Soluble Components that Interact with Serum. Bacterial endotoxin

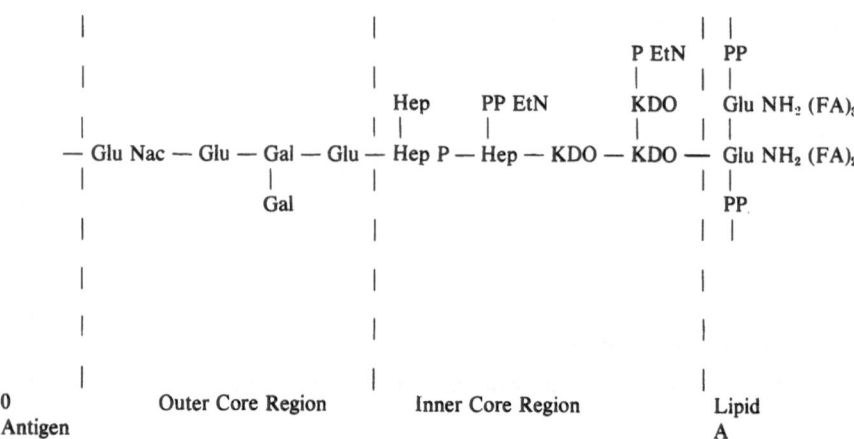

FIG. 5.11. The structure of bacterial endotoxin [after Westphal *et al., J. Infect. Dis.* **128**(Suppl.) (1973).] The lipid A backbone is a disaccharide unit of two β-6-D-glucosamine residues linked by 1,4-pyrophosphate groups. Both glucosamine molecules are substituted with fatty acids on each available carbon atom and in the amino group. The fatty acid on the amino groups is usually β-hydroxymyristic acid. Linked to one of the glucosamine units is the inner polysaccharide core. The outer core is composed of a pentasaccharide unit, and attached to the outer core are the repeating 3- and 4-sugar units of the 0 antigen. 0 antigens vary from one organism to another, but the outer and inner core regions and lipid A are similar or identical for large groups of bacteria. [KDO: ketodeoxyoctonate (an 8-carbon sugar); EtN: ethanolamine; Hep: L-glycero-D-mannoheptose (a 7-carbon sugar); Glu: glucose; Glu NAc: *N*-acetyl glucosamine; Gal: galactose; FA: fatty acid.]

is a structural component of all gram-negative organisms, and is liberated into the medium in low concentrations wherever they are growing. The molecule contains three domains; the major portion is carbohydrate, and is identical with the O antigen of the parent strain. This portion is covalently linked to a basal region that is very similar for all gram-negative organisms, and this region in turn is linked to a glycolipid, lipid A (Fig. 5.11). Lipid A is responsible for the toxic effects of the molecule; in addition, it can cause the fixation of complement components by the alternate pathway. All normal human sera contain antibody against the basal region, and many contain low levels of antibody against O antigens. Most of these antibodies are of the IgM class, and are very efficient at fixing complement by the classic pathway. Thus, if endotoxin is allowed access to serum, complement is fixed by one or another pathway, and chemotactic factors will be generated.

Many other soluble bacterial products are antigenic, and antibodies to them exist in normal sera. For example, over 30 different antibodies to components in streptococcal culture filtrates can be demonstrated in pooled, concentrated human sera. Similarly, almost everyone has preformed antibody to the staphylococcal α toxin. These antibodies develop as a consequence of exposure to the organisms when they colonize one or another of the body surfaces, often without any overt evidence of disease. All these products would thus be expected to develop chemotactic activity when exposed to serum.

Ward has also shown that several extracellular bacterial proteases can generate chemotactic activity by cleaving C3 or C5, or both.

(iii) Interaction of Bacterial Bodies with Serum. Washed, dead bacteria are not chemotactic when tested in the absence of serum by membrane techniques. That they are not is only to be expected: Since the organisms are dead, they can produce no soluble factors of their own; since serum is not present, no complement components can be activated; and since the neutrophils do not have access to the bacteria, no neutrophil-derived factors can come into play. However, all dead bacteria are chemotactic when serum is present in the system. In part, this is attributable to low levels of antibody against bacterial components. All bacterial cell walls have a basal layer of peptidoglycan that provides structural support for the cell membrane and is responsible for the bacterial shape. Nonpathogenic gram-positive organisms expose this layer to the environment; since all humans are colonized with bacteria, all have antibody against peptidoglycan. Other structural components held in common by large classes of bacteria are the teichoic acids in gram-positive organisms and the endotoxins in gram-negative organisms.

Pathogenic organisms usually have outer layers that cover the cell wall components that would make them vulnerable, and present the host with a new surface, specific for the organism concerned. Sometimes this outer layer is thick and easily visible; it is then called a *capsule*. Sometimes it is visible only in electron micrographs; a good example is the M protein layer of *Streptococcus pyogenes*. Capsules are usually made of carbohydrate, and one group of a few sugar residues is monotonously repeated all over the bacterial surface. The monotony is an important safety device; unless the host has exactly the right antibody available, he will have to make it from scratch.

Complement is most efficiently fixed by antibody; however, even pathogenic bacteria for which no trace of antibody can be detected can nonetheless fix complement by the alternate pathway. This will lead to generation of the same chemotactic factors as if the complement had been fixed by antibody.

(iv) and (v). Chemotactic Factors from Neutrophils. We have already noted in passing that neutrophils generate chemotactic factors when they phagocytose organisms. One such factor is prostaglandin E_1; another is the factor investigated by Zigmond and Hirsch, which seemed to be a protein. Both these factors appear to be generated efficiently in the absence of complement. In addition, the proteolytic enzymes of neutrophil granules can cleave complement components, with the release of chemotactic fragments (see below).

It is thus easy to see why bacteria are chemotactic no matter how one does the experiment. Naturally, the precise contribution of each particular mechanism will vary from one experimental setup to another, and of course it is impossible to assess from this kind of evidence how "important" individual factors are *in vivo*.

(b) The Complement System. Complement has been mentioned at several points previously, but has not been discussed *per se*. It is the common name for a group of at least 11 proteins that are found in the normal serum of man and animals. It was discovered by Bordet, who was interested in the lysis of gram-negative bacteria by serum. He found that the lytic activity could be divided into two components. One was specific for the particular organism and was stable to moderate heat at 56°C; this component subsequently turned out to be antibody. The other was nonspecific and would lyse any organism that had antibody on its surface; this component was "complementary" to antibody, and was therefore called *complement*. It was destroyed by heating to 56°C for 30 min.

Complement has become steadily more complicated, and many details of its action remain to be worked out.[28] It has now become clear that there are two separate mechanisms for complement activation, the classical and the alternate pathways.

(i) The Classical Pathway. The classical pathway was discovered first, and the proteins in it can conveniently be divided into three groups. The first is the recognition unit, which recognizes antigen–antibody complexes, whether the antigen be a soluble protein or part of a bacterium or eukaryotic cell. The second is concerned with the assembly of an enzymatically active complex. Once assembled, the complex acts on a component of the third group, which is concerned with the actual destruction of bacteria and

foreign cells, and is known as the *attack mechanism*. As the different complement proteins were discovered, they were assigned numbers, and in general the numerical sequence indicates the order in which they react. However, since component C4 was discovered before the mechanism had been worked out, it is out of order, and reacts directly after C1. Cells that have fixed complement components are described by a shorthand nomenclature, as follows: *S* (for antibody-combining Site) *A* (because Antibody is required for classical complement fixation) C1, 4, 2, 3, 5, 6, 7, 8, 9. Cells that have reacted with only some of the components may form more or less stable intermediates; an SAC1423 cell is one that has reacted with the first four components.

The Recognition Unit. The classical pathway is triggered by the presence of antibody on the bacterial surface. Antigen binds to antibody molecules in the Fab regions, but an allosteric change occurs that results in the exposure of previously hidden determinants in the Fc region. This region then binds C1, which is the recognition protein for the classical pathway. Not all antigen–antibody complexes can bind C1; IgA and IgE complexes are ineffective, as are some of the subclasses of IgG. The most effective antibody is IgM; one molecule of bound IgM suffices to fix complement. Fixation by IgG demands that two molecules of bound IgG lie close together. When the antigen is in free solution, there is no great difference in the efficiency of complement fixation by IgG and IgM; because antigen molecules can diffuse together, cross-links can form, and a lattice, and ultimately a macroscopically visible precipitate, can build up. However, when the antigen is a bacterium, the antigenic determinants are held rigidly apart because they are structurally part of the bacterial cell wall or capsule. Since a single bacterium may have many thousands of identical determinants on its outer surface, it is very improbable that two IgG molecules will lie adjacent in a manner that will allow complement fixation to occur (Fig. 5.12). For this reason, IgG is effective on a bacterial surface only when a great deal of antibody is available and the whole surface can be covered with IgG. IgM, which binds complement when only one molecule fixes to antigen, is thus at an enormous advantage, because one antibody molecule can lead to the destruction of one bacterium.

Assembly of an Enzymatically Active Complex. C1 is actually a complex of three proteins, C1q, C1r, and C1s, that are held together by noncovalent bonds. The most important binding mechanism is ionic bonding through calcium ions, because chelating agents such as EDTA allow the

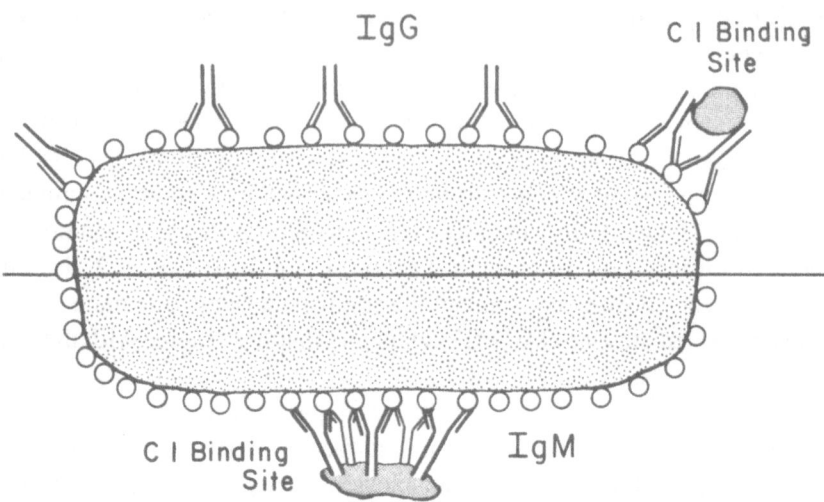

FIG. 5.12. A hypothetical bacterial cell bearing a single immunodeterminant repeated many times. Above the line are six bound IgG molecules; only the two on the right can fix complement. Below the line is a single bound IgM molecule; it shows the typical crablike shape with all five of its pentamers attached, and can fix complement by itself.

three components to separate. The recognition protein, which binds to fixed antibody, is C1q. C1s is an esterase that becomes activated when the C1 complex becomes fixed. The function of C1r is not known in detail, but it is thought to mediate the activation of C1s on receiving a signal from C1q. The enzymatic activity of C1s can be measured with several synthetic esters, but its natural substrate is C4. The pattern of the reaction is repeated throughout the complement sequence; C4 is split into a large fragment, C4b, which attaches to the bacterial surface, and a small fragment, C4a, which drifts off into the solution. C4b now adsorbs C2, which is also split by C1s. One fragment, C2a, remains bound to the C4b; another, C2b, is lost into the fluid phase. The bacterium now has C1q, r, and s, C4b, and C2a bound on its surface in proximity. C4b and C2a together form a new enzyme, symbolized as $\overline{C4b,2a}$, which can cleave the next component, C3. Again, two fragments are formed; the large C3b binds to the bacterial surface, and the smaller C3a remains in solution. And again a new enzyme is created, this time involving three large complement component fragments and known as $\overline{C4b,2a,3b}$. This enzyme is the one that activates the attack mechanism (Fig. 5.13). Only one C3b molecule is required to make the enzyme $\overline{C4b,2a,3b}$; however, a single $\overline{4b,2a}$ complex splits many C3 molecules, and the bacterial surface may bind C3b fragments at sites far removed from the $\overline{4b,2a}$ complex that formed them. These fragments are unable to cleave C5, but are important opsonins (see Chapter 6).

The Attack Mechanism. The attack mechanism is initiated when the assembled enzyme $\overline{C4b,2a,3b}$ cleaves C5 into a large fragment, C5b, and a smaller fragment, C5a. From this point on, complement components are not cleaved, but assemble themselves into macromolecular complexes by noncovalent forces. C5b is unstable: If it remains bound to C3b, its half-life is about 8 min; if it is released into the fluid phase, its half-life is only a fraction of a second. If C6 is available, the two proteins combine, and the complex is stable whether on a cell membrane or in the fluid phase. The C5b,6 complex now adsorbs C7 to make the soluble trimolecular complex C5b,6,7. This complex is very unstable unless it can bind to a lipid membrane, but the decay process does not appear to involve splitting a fragment off any of the components. Because of the instability of the 5b,6,7 complex, it is much more likely to succeed in binding to a cell membrane if the 5b component is held near the membrane by C3b. Cell lysis by fluid phase C5b,6,7 is possible, but is so improbable that it occurs only in the presence of huge amounts of complement components. If the 5b,6,7, complex does bind to a cell membrane, the addition of C8 and C9 will cause that cell to lyse.

From the point of view of the neutrophil, the proteins that mediate the final attack on the cell membrane and lead to lysis are irrelevant. Bacteriolysis is in any case confined to gram-negative organisms; gram-positive organisms become a little sticky and may clump together when acted on by complement, but their vitality is unimpaired. Gram-positive organisms are therefore disposed of entirely by phagocytosis, and it seems probable that few gram-negative organisms remain at liberty long enough for complement-mediated lysis to occur.

(ii) The Alternate Pathway. The alternate pathway of complement fixation was discovered by Pillemer in the 1950s, but only in the last ten years has there been general agreement about its existence and importance. Pillemer thought that a single substance, which he named *properdin,* was responsible for the activity.[29] It is now clear that the pathway is complex, but the number of components and the nature and order of their reactions are still under active investigation, and the following account is provisional. This pathway is activated by all immunoglobulins that bind antigen; furthermore, it can be shown that the Fab fragment, not the Fc, is responsible for the activation. It is possible to partially digest immunoglobulin G with pepsin, so that the Fc portion is split off and the two Fab regions are left

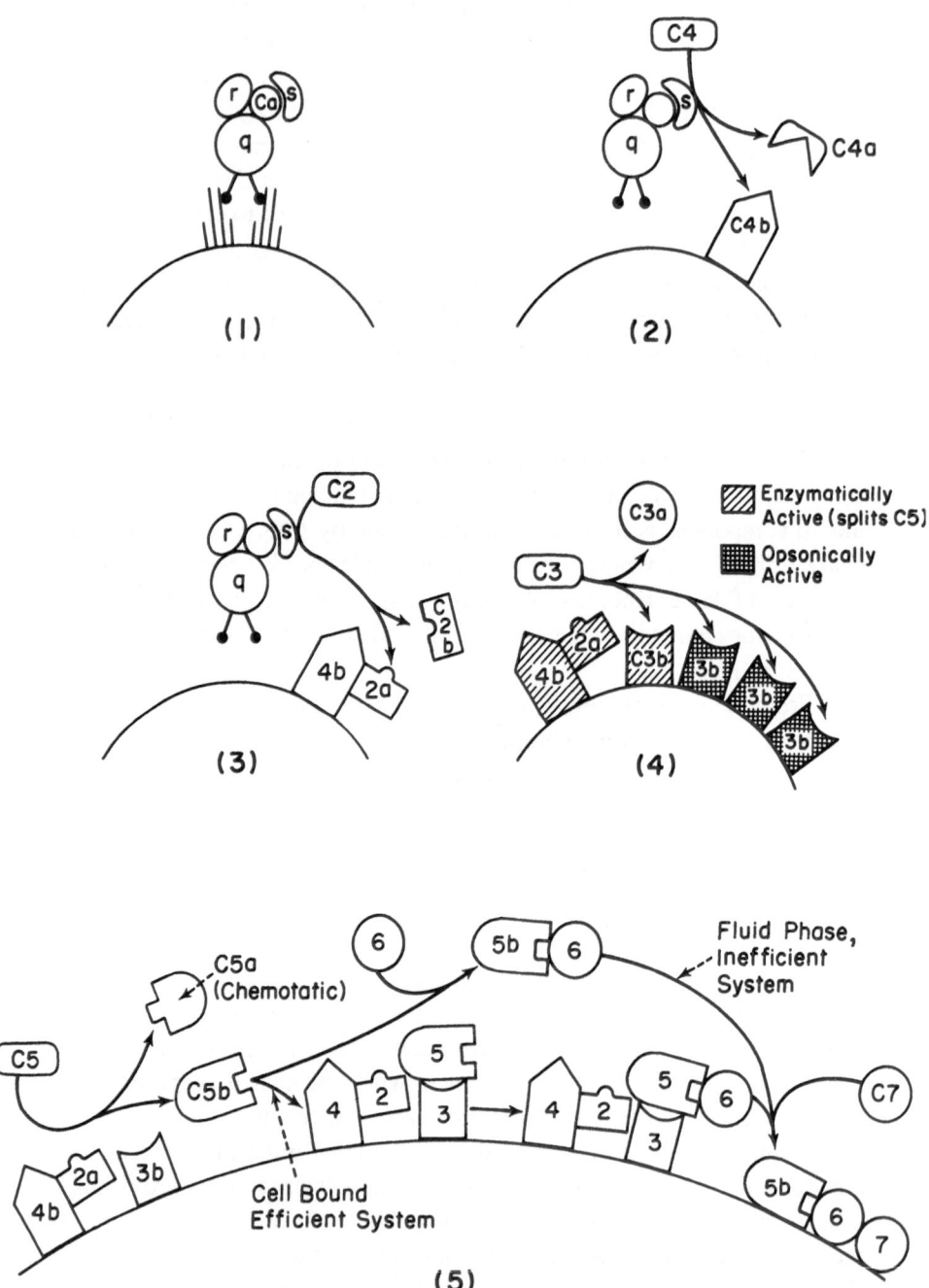

linked by a single sulfhydryl bond. This dimer is known as F(ab')$_2$ to distinguish it from the monovalent Fab piece obtained by digestion with papain. Since F(ab')$_2$ is divalent, aggregation, lattices, and precipitates can develop; these fix complement by the alternate pathway. The alternate pathway is also activated by bacterial products, notably endotoxin, and by certain carbohydrates such as the cell walls of yeasts and the capsules of pneumococci. It is not known whether traces of antibody are necessary for the initiation of the alternate pathway; certainly, if antibody is required, the quantity is unmeasurable by present methods. However, antibody does potentiate complement fixation by the alternate pathway.

The C3-cleaving enzyme in the alternate pathway contains two new components, factor B and factor D, and the same C3b complement component that we have already met in the classical pathway. It appears that the first step in the assembly requires the presence of a small quantity of C3b fixed on the bacterial surface. Since C3b is a cleavage product of the normal serum protein C3, there arises at once the question how the C3b is generated. No precise answer can be given; there are several proteolytic enzyme systems in plasma that could potentially cleave a little C3; for example, if bacteria activated the Hageman factor, one would expect the generation of small quantities of plasmin and kallikrein. It is possible that a certain amount of C3 is constantly broken down under normal circumstances; a patient is known who appears to lack a regulator protein that destroys newly formed C3b. This man constantly turns over his alternate pathway, and consumes so much C3 and factor B that he is unable to synthesize enough to replace the losses.

At any rate, given a small quantity of C3b fixed to the bacterial surface, factor B is adsorbed and is cleaved by factor D. Factor D is activated by another component, properdin. The assembled enzyme $\overline{\text{DBC3b}}$ is able to

---

FIG. 5.13. Assembly of classical complement components on a cell surface. (1) C1q has a central portion with several radiating arms that make contact with bound antibody. (ii, iii) The activated C1s cleaves C4 and C2 successively; C4b binds to the cell membrane, C2a binds to C4b. (iv) C4b,2a cleaves C3; one molecule will bind locally to give the $\overline{4\text{b,2a,3b}}$ complex, but hundreds of C3b molecules may bind all over the cell surface and opsonize it (Chapter 6). (v) The $\overline{4\text{b,2a,3b}}$ complex cleaves C5; C5a is chemotactic, C5b decays rapidly unless C6 is available to stabilize it. If C5b remains bound to C3b, it decays more slowly than if it is released into the fluid phase. Bound C5b molecules thus have a better chance of finding a C6 molecule to stabilize them. When C7 is added, cell bound $\overline{\text{C5b,67}}$ complexes will be near the membrane, and are more likely to insert into it before they decay.

cleave C3. The process is therefore autocatalytic, because newly generated C3b can fix to bacterial surfaces and initiate another cycle.

Other components for the properdin pathway must certainly exist, and a number of interactions with the classical pathway confuse the situation still further. The properdin pathway proceeds normally in the presence of antibody against C2, which completely blocks the classical pathway. However, the properdin pathway is greatly slowed in serum of guinea pigs congenitally deficient in C4, and the defect is reversed by adding C4. The C4 is clearly not acting as it does in the classical pathway, where its role is to cleave C2, and how it does work is unknown.

The alternate pathway enzyme that cleaves C5 contains C3b, factor B, and factor D, but it differs from the C3-cleaving enzyme in its stability; hence, there must be some additional component as yet unrecognized. As far as we know, the cleavages of C3 and C5 that are induced by the alternate pathway enzymes are identical with those of the classical pathway enzymes, and the biological activities of the small fragments C3a and C5a are identical.

(iii) The C5b,6,7 Complex. The first workers to attempt to assign to particular complement components the chemotactic activity that developed when antigen–antibody precipitates were incubated in serum were Ward, Cochrane, and Müller-Eberhard.[30] They showed that in normal rabbit and human sera treated with antigen–antibody complexes, chemotactic activity seemed to be associated with a trimolecular complex of C5, C6, and C7. This complex was originally shown by Pevikon block electrophoresis, but in a subsequent paper, was also demonstrated by sucrose density gradient centrifugation. They also showed that a similar chemotactic activity appeared in the serum of rabbits injected with aggregated gamma globulin, or with zymosan, a carbohydrate preparation from yeast cell wall. Using human complement components assembled on sheep red cells, they found that the major chemotactic activity was not generated until C7 had been added. It may be worth noting that the C5b,6,7 complex has been associated with chemotaxis only by inference; it has not been isolated in a pure state, as have the C5 and C3 fragments discussed below. Parenthetically, fluid phase C5b,6,7 complex is unable to attach to cell surfaces, and is therefore hemolytically inactive (compare the rapid decay of C5b,6,7 complex above).

(iv) The C5a Fragment. While the C5b,6,7 complex certainly does exist and is probably chemotactic, the smaller fragment, C5a, is also chemotactic and does not require either C6 or C7 for its activity. Shin and

his colleagues reacted sheep erythrocytes sequentially with antibody and functionally purified guinea pig complement components.[31] Functional purity means that 10,000 hemolytic units of a particular complement component contained less than 1 unit of any other component, though noncomplement proteins might be present. Assembly of complexes SAC1,4,2,3b with liberation of C3a into the fluid phase did not give rise to chemotactic activity. When SAC1,4,2,3b complexes were treated with C5 and were then centrifuged, chemotactic activity was found in the supernate. By the use of C5 labeled with ^{125}I, it was possible to show that the original C5 molecule with a sedimentation constant of 7.8S had been split into two components, 7.45 S and 1.5 S. The smaller fragment attracted neutrophils in a Boyden chamber, and also caused liberation of histamine from guinea pig ileum. The active fragment appeared to be homogeneous, as judged by gel filtration on Sephadex G-75 and by electrophoresis on both 7.5 and 15% acrylamide gels at acid pH. In all these experiments, chemotactic and histamine-liberating activity coincided with the radioactively labeled 1.5 S fragment.

Recent work by Clark, Frank, and Kimball has suggested that two chemotactic fragments of C5 may be liberated when antigen–antibody complexes interact with human serum: one of molecular weight about 10,000 daltons and the other about 17,000 daltons.[32] It was possible to resolve the two by chromatography on Sephadex G-100. If C5 was radiolabeled, both fragments were labeled, and the chemotactic activity of both was abolished by antibody against C5. Either the classic or the alternate pathway could generate these fragments. Presumably, in the experiments of Shin and Snyderman (below), these two components were not resolved, although it is also possible that a species difference is involved, and that human serum proteases were responsible for the cleavage of C5a seen in Clark's experiments.

Snyderman provided evidence that the small fragment or fragments of C5 are important chemotactic agents *in vivo*.[33] The experimental model selected for study was the inflammatory response that results when shellfish glycogen is injected into the peritoneal cavity. He used the normal guinea pig, and C5-deficient and normal mice. In the guinea pig, he found that measurable chemotactic activity was present in the peritoneal fluid 30 min after injection of glycogen, and that it reached a maximum at 1–2 hr. Most of the activity migrated on Sephadex G-100 with an apparent molecular weight of about 15,000, and it was neutralized by antibody to C5. In the mice, it was shown that treatment of serum with antigen–antibody complexes or with endotoxin caused liberation of chemotactic activity from normal mouse serum, but not from C5-deficient serum. Inflammatory responses in the mouse peritoneum were induced by injection of endotoxin. In normal animals, neutrophil accumulation was obvious by 3 hr, and analysis of the fluid for chemotactic activity showed that it was maximal at 1 hr and remained demonstrable for at least 12 hr. Gel filtration confirmed that most of the activity was due to a 15,000-dalton fragment. In C5-deficient mice, chemotactic activity in the fluid was negligible until 24 hr after the endotoxin injection; correspondingly, neutrophils were very sparse until 24–48 hr. At 24 hr, 7 times more neutrophils could be recovered from the peritoneal cavity of normal mice than from C5-deficient mice.

This evidence establishes that C5a is an important chemotactic agent in at least some types of inflammatory response. It is curious that the C5-deficient mouse is not noticeably prone to infection and can be housed in normal animal-care facilities without undue mortality from infectious disease. Presumably, this immunity means that under most circumstances, other pathways can attract neutrophils into the tissues. However, there is one paper showing a difference in the mortality produced in normal and C5-deficient mice by an experimental infection. This was an intravenous challenge of mice with the Type 25 pneumococcus; the LD_{50} for normal mice was about 10 times greater than that for C5-deficient mice.

There is also evidence that C5 deficiency is important in humans. Families are known in which some members have a C5 protein that is biologically inactive, although it does react with antibody to C5. The proband was discovered because of a succession of bacterial infections.

(v) C3 Fragments. It is generally agreed that the fragmentation of C3 that occurs during complement fixation does not lead to the generation of chemotactic activity. However, Ward has convincingly shown that proteolytic enzymes can lead to the generation of chemotactic C3 fragments, and that these are important in certain situations *in vivo*.

Ward's initial experiments involved partial digestion of C3 with plasmin, a proteolytic enzyme that is activated from an inactive precursor during blood clotting. The active fragment of C3 had a molecular weight of about 6000, as judged by gel filtration. Subsequent work showed that other proteolytic enzymes, such as trypsin, could generate chemotactic activity from C3; one of the more interesting findings was that the proteolytic enzymes of neutrophil lysosomes could do likewise. Subsequently, Hill and Ward demonstrated that many tissues contain proteases, active at a neutral pH, that can cleave C3 and generate a small chemotactic fragment. This, then, is the probable explanation of the results of Ryan and Hurley quoted earlier; if tissue is killed by an inflammatory stimulus, its neutral proteases will be released, which will hydrolyze C3, and chemotaxis will be observed. This explanation also fits some curious results of Bessis: He was watching neutrophils wander at random over a glass slide, and killed one instantaneously with a laser beam. Its companions immediately converged on the dead cell and ate it. However, Bessis noted that if a fragment of the dead cell floated off into the medium, it was ignored and even pushed aside by new arrivals. This strongly suggests that the chemotactic activity was generated indirectly.

Hill and Ward provided conclusive evidence that chemotactic factors generated from C3 by dead tissue are important *in vivo*.[34] If an artery is blocked, naturally or experimentally, the tissue that it supplies dies unless arterial blood can find its way around by some alternative channel. Such a volume of dead tissue is called an *infarct*, and a characteristic feature of infarcts is that after two or three days, they develop a dense infiltrate of neutrophils around the edges. It is possible to deplete a rat of virtually all its C3 by injecting it with a purified protein from cobra venom. Hill and Ward produced myocardial infarcts in rats by tying the left coronary artery, and showed that rats depleted of C3 did not develop the usual neutrophil infiltrates around their infarcts.

Ward and Zvaifler applied this knowledge of chemotactic fragments of C3 and C5 to the pathogenesis of human arthritis.[35] Much of the damage in arthritis of all types is thought to result from digestion of articular cartilage by neutrophil enzymes. In rheumatoid arthritis, it is probable that antigen–antibody reactions occur within the joint cavity; accordingly, one would expect to find the C5-dependent factors, C5a and C5,6,7, in the joint fluid. Other arthritides are due to direct damage to joint tissue by trauma, infections, and other insults. Under these circumstances, one might expect to find C3 fragments generated by tissue proteases. Ward and Zvaifler confirmed these expectations, and further showed that the joint fluid in gout contained a proteolytic enzyme that generated chemotactic activity from C3. Once neutrophils have entered a joint cavity, or any other inflammatory site, the proteolytic enzymes in their lysosomes will be partially released during phagocytosis. Ward and Zvaifler showed that these enzymes could generate chemotactic activity from C5 as well as C3. Thus, chemotactic fragments would continue to summon neutrophils until there was nothing left to phagocytose.

(c) Other Chemotactic Proteins and Protein Fragments. Wilkinson
has recently suggested that the chemotactic activity generated by cleavages
of C3 and C5 is merely an example of a general phenomenon.[36] Many
proteins become chemotactic when subjected to mild proteolysis or to
denaturation. The most impressive example of the latter effect is provided
by hemoglobin. This protein is not chemotactic in its native state, but if the
heme moiety is removed, the globin remnant becomes so. Addition of free
heme allows the molecule to resume its original shape, and the chemotactic
activity disappears. Myoglobin behaves similarly. It was hypothesized that
the crucial factor that made proteins chemotactic was a partial loss of
secondary and tertiary structure, so that hydrophobic residues that normally faced the interior of the molecule became exposed. This hypothesis
was tested directly by substituting chemical groups of various types into
human serum albumin: Nonpolar groups made it chemotactic; polar ones
did not.

Chemotactic fragments are liberated during blood clotting; clotting is
always accompanied by local fibrinolysis. The cleavage of fibrinogen by
plasmin causes the liberation of fibrinopeptides; fibrinopeptide B has
recently been shown to be chemotactic, while fibrinopeptides A, AP, and
AY are not.[37] In the process of kinin generation, kallikrein is formed from
an inactive precursor, and in addition to its kinin-generating action, it
appears to be chemotactic.[38] Perhaps the most impressive evidence for the
importance *in vivo* of a noncomplement-derived protein was obtained by
Yoshinaga and his colleagues.[39] They induced passive Arthus reactions in
rabbit skin by injecting anti-BSA intravenously, followed by BSA intrader-
mally. The lesions were excised, frozen, sliced, and extracted with ace-
tone. The acetone-insoluble material was then extracted into phosphate
buffer, and a 50% ammonium sulfate cut was taken. The precipitate proved
to contain a strongly chemotactic agent, which differed from most other
such agents in that it had little or no effect on vascular permeability. An
identical agent was isolated from burned skin. By successive chromatography on DEAE Sephadex, CM Sephadex, and G-200 Sephadex, they were
able to obtain an active material that was homogeneous, as judged by
acrylamide gel electrophoresis at two different pH's and by sedimentation
velocity in the analytical ultracentrifuge. The material proved to be a
fragment of immunoglobulin G, with a molecular weight of approximately
140,000. It gave single bands when run against antirabbit serum in Ouchterlony gels or in immunoelectrophoresis, and these bands gave reactions of
identity with known rabbit IgG bands. They were able to form the chemo-

tactically active fragment of IgG *in vitro* by digesting IgG with a protease found in most tissues and in both neutrophils and histiocytes. When the fragment was injected into rabbit skin, it stimulated palisading of neutrophils on venule walls and their subsequent emigration between endothelial cells. Since there was no increased vascular permeability, one must suppose that the neutrophils forced the endothelial cells apart, and that the gaps closed behind them.

(d) Prostaglandins. Another complement-independent chemotactic substance is prostaglandin E_1. We saw above that it is probably responsible for the delayed phase of increased vascular permeability, and Kaley discovered that in Boyden chambers, it is chemotactic at a concentration of 1 μg/ml. It must therefore contribute to the emigration of neutrophils during the delayed phase.[40]

There are thus a very large number of mechanisms by which chemotactic agents could conceivably develop in injured or infected tissue. However, while it may be true that leukocytes respond to hydrophobic amino acid residues, only those protein splits that are biologically plausible need be considered further. Complement components, prekallikrein, and immunoglobulin occur naturally, and during inflammation, they demonstrably undergo changes that render them chemotactic. It is not probable that hemoglobin is commonly robbed of its heme *in vivo*.

5.2.5. The Serine Esterase of Neutrophil Membranes

Becker has discovered that a number of different chemotactic agents seem to share a common pathway when acting on the neutrophil, in that they cause activation of an esterase on the neutrophil surface.[41] This esterase contains a serine residue in its active site, and is therefore susceptible to inactivation by diisopropylfluorophosphate and certain phosphonates. Neutrophils incubated with these inhibitors are unable to give a chemotactic response either to complement components or to bacterial chemotactic factors. The esterase is normally inactive, but measurable activity develops when the cell is exposed to C3 or C5 fragments. Once the cell has responded to any one complement component, it is unable to respond again either to the same component or to any other stimulus, apparently because the serine esterase has a short half-life, and cannot be regenerated once it has decayed. Exposure to a complement component is therefore one mechanism for immobilizing neutrophils once they have arrived at an inflammatory site. However, cells unable to give a chemotactic response are still perfectly adequate at phagocytosing and killing microorganisms. Bacterial chemotactic factors differ in that they appear to activate the esterase only in one localized part of the cell, and sequential responses to bacterial factors are possible. Once the esterase has been activated all over the cell, however, bacterial factors cannot induce a chemotactic response. This is why bacterial factors are ineffective when the neutrophil has responded to a complement fragment. That sequential responses to bacterial factors are possible is one reason why chemotaxis of neutrophils toward bacteria is so easy to demonstrate.

5.2.6. Neutrophil-Immobilizing Factors

Another factor that immobilizes neutrophils was described by Goetzl and Austen.[42] Actually, they described three such factors—one liberated from neutrophils when they phagocytose bacteria, one when they were stimulated with endotoxin, and a third when they were exposed to a pH of 5.0 for an hour. However, there was no hard evidence that these factors really differed from one another. They appeared to be small proteins of molecular weight about 8000 daltons. The neutrophils were not killed, merely immobilized, and they remained effective phagocytes. Obviously, it might be biologically useful if a neutrophil that had phagocytosed one organism liberated substances that held other neutrophils in the vicinity.

5.3. Antagonists of Inflammation

So far, we have discussed only mechanisms that tend to increase the inflammatory response. Some are autocatalytic, and those that are not tend to mutually enhance and reinforce one another. Histamine causes increased vascular permeability, which allows serum proteins to leak into the area, which allows complement components to interact with bacteria, which generates fragments that increase vascular permeability and attract neutrophils. Neutrophils exposed to bacteria liberate substances that attract more neutrophils, and so on. However, an excessive degree of inflammatory response leads to destruction of host tissue. This destruction is perhaps most clearly seen in the Arthus reaction. If one injects horse serum into the skin of a rabbit, nothing happens. The serum is thus harmless in and of itself. However, if one injects the serum once weekly for an extended period, one first sees a response of local swelling and erythema, and ultimately hemorrhagic necrosis of the skin occurs after each injection.

What has happened is that the rabbit has developed precipitating antibody to one or more horse serum proteins, so that antigen–antibody complexes form locally in the injection site. These complexes fix complement, chemotactic factors are generated, neutrophils emigrate into the area, and hemorrhagic necrosis ensues as the result of digestion of blood vessel walls by proteolytic enzymes from neutrophil granules. Since the serum itself was innocuous, this severe destructive response results entirely from overactivity of the responses of the host.

It is essential that any response capable of such violent activity be well provided with mechanisms that tend to shut it off. The primary mechanism is the removal of the noxious stimulus. For example, once all the bacteria in an inflammatory site have been phagocytosed, generation of chemotactic factors will virtually cease. Natural antagonists of most inflammatory mediators are known: There are enzymes in normal tissue that inactivate histamine, serotonin, and bradykinin; normal serum contains proteins that antagonize C1, C2, C4, C3, and C6, and another that destroys C3a and C5a; antagonists of many different types of proteolytic enzymes exist in serum and in normal tissues.

Several children are known who are unusually susceptible to bacterial infections, apparently because their serum contains proteins that act directly on neutrophils to render them insensitive to chemotactic stimuli. If the patient's neutrophils were washed and suspended in normal serum, they responded normally, and if normal neutrophils were put into the patient's serum, they became unable to respond.[43] Another group of patients appears to have higher than normal levels of a protein or proteins that destroy C5a and C5b67. Most of these patients have been adults with Laennec's cirrhosis or Hodgkin's disease, and while in both cases there are clearly multiple factors predisposing to infection, it is possible that lack of chemotactic stimuli in local lesions contributes.

5.4. Summary

The cardinal features of inflammation are vasodilatation, increased vascular permeability, and the emigration of phagocytic cells from blood into injured tissue. These processes are caused by local hormones released from injured cells, or generated by the cleavage of serum proteins. It is possible that direct injury to vessel walls is also important. The initial increase in vascular permeability occurs within minutes of injury and lasts about ½ hr; it is mediated by the release of histamine and serotonin from mast cells. A delayed phase of increased vascular permeability begins about 1 hr after injury and lasts for an extended period. This phase is initially mediated by the generation of bradykinin by serum kallikrein, but the most important mediators seem to be prostaglandins synthesized either by injured tissue cells or by the invading phagocytes. All these substances cause the development of gaps between endothelial cells, through which serum proteins and phagocytes can pass into the tissue.

Several substances that attract neutrophils and monocytes are generated in inflammatory sites; their relative importance varies according to circumstances. Activation of complement by either the classic or the alternate pathway leads to cleavage of C5; the small C5a fragment is directly chemotactic, and the large C5b fragment is chemotactic in at least some species when combined with C6 and C7. Chemotactic fragments can be generated from C3 by the action of serum, tissue, bacterial, or neutrophil proteases. Bacteria are chemotactic because they have several ways of activating complement components, and because they produce small proteins that are directly chemotactic. In sterile inflammations, prostaglandins are likely to be important chemotactic agents, and a fragment of IgG is at least partially responsible for the neutrophil accumulation in Arthus reactions.

Once neutrophils have been attracted into tissue by any of the substances named above, phagocytosis triggers the release from neutrophils of substances that attract neutrophils. Phagocytosis also causes the release of a neutrophil-immobilizing hormone, so that neutrophils already in the tissue cannot wander away. The net result of all this activity is that neutrophils will continue to accumulate in injured tissue until there is nothing left to phagocytose.

Much less is known about mechanisms that shut off the inflammatory response. Normal serum contains enzymes that destroy histamine and kinins, and proteins that antagonize the activated forms of several complement components. It also contains proteins that inhibit the proteolytic enzymes that are generated in inflamed tissue and that unchecked would lead to the exponential generation of more and more inflammatory mediators. The details of this sytem of checks and balances are not understood.

Selected Reading

Zweifach, B. W., Grant, L., and McCluskey, R. T. (eds.), *The Inflammatory Response*, 2nd ed., 3 volumes, Academic Press, New York, 1973–1974.

6

Phagocytosis

It was well established before 1910 that phagocytosis is one of the main defenses against bacterial infection, and that neutrophils are aided in taking up bacteria by antibody and complement. Progress since then has consisted largely of filling in the details, and while a good deal of phenomenological information has accumulated, we are still far from being able to give a complete account of the process.

As in chemotaxis, there are substantial difficulties with the experimental methods. Neutrophils may be obtained either from the blood or from inflammatory exudates. Isolation of neutrophils from blood always involves unphysiological manipulations, and the effect of procedures such as exposure to distilled water for 30 sec is impossible to evaluate. We also have little idea of how neutrophils are affected by the events that are set in train as soon as blood is exposed to a foreign surface. Activation of the Hageman factor, or degranulation of platelets, liberates powerful inflammatory mediators that are known to affect neutrophil behavior. Neutrophils isolated from peritoneal exudates have left the blood vessels in response to chemotactic stimuli that are known to change their behavior permanently, and have been exposed for some hours to inflammatory mediators of all types. Clear differences between blood neutrophils and exudate neutrophils can be easily demonstrated, yet cells from both sources are usually supposed to be comparable, and normal. The media in which the cells are suspended vary in crucial parameters such as pH, ionic strength, and divalent cation concentration. The concentration of cells varies from one experiment to another. Everyone uses a different organism, different strains of the same organism, or even nonliving particles such as carbon or starch. The cell:particle ratio varies, as does the time of incubation. Serum is added in various concentrations, and with or without heat inactivation. It is not uncommon to review an experiment performed with the cells of one species, antibody from a second, and complement from a third. Until recently, phagocytosis was measured by making smears, staining bacteria and phagocytes, and counting either the number of cells that had ingested one or more particles or the number of particles per cell. Each method had its proponents, but either was tedious and difficult. Indirect methods are usually based on counting the surviving bacteria at given times, but the precise relationship of the counts to the phagocytosis of organisms is often in doubt. Other indirect methods measure effects of phagocytosis on the neutrophils, such as increased hexose monophosphate shunt activity or nitro blue tetrazolium reduction. With these methods, it is known that the variables measured are affected by both the type and the number of particles ingested, and it is not clear what is being measured.

The upshot of all this variability is that experiments on phagocytosis are strictly relative. The late Dr. W. Barry Wood, Jr., once remarked to me that he could rig a phagocytic experiment to get any result he wanted. If one was interested in demonstrating the opsonic power of IgG, one used glass tubes, in which there was little or no spontaneous phagocytosis. If one was interested in the opsonic power of C3b, one diluted the cell suspension a little more, and kept the gamma globulin concentration down, so that now there was little or no phagocytosis until C3 was added. Clearly, it makes no sense under these circumstances to claim that a particular substance is "required" for phagocytosis to occur. It helps or hinders, and that is all that can be said. Furthermore, as Wood showed, neutrophils in living animals have resources available to them that are not apparent *in vitro*. The true significance of a mechanism can therefore be evaluated only in living animals.

6.1. Mechanisms of Phagocytosis

6.1.1. General Considerations

The most crucial fact about phagocytosis is that when the organism is once attached to the cell membrane, pseudopods pass around each side of it, meet, and then fuse together (Fig. 6.1). The bacterium is enclosed in a pouch of cell membrane, the inner layer of which was originally the outer

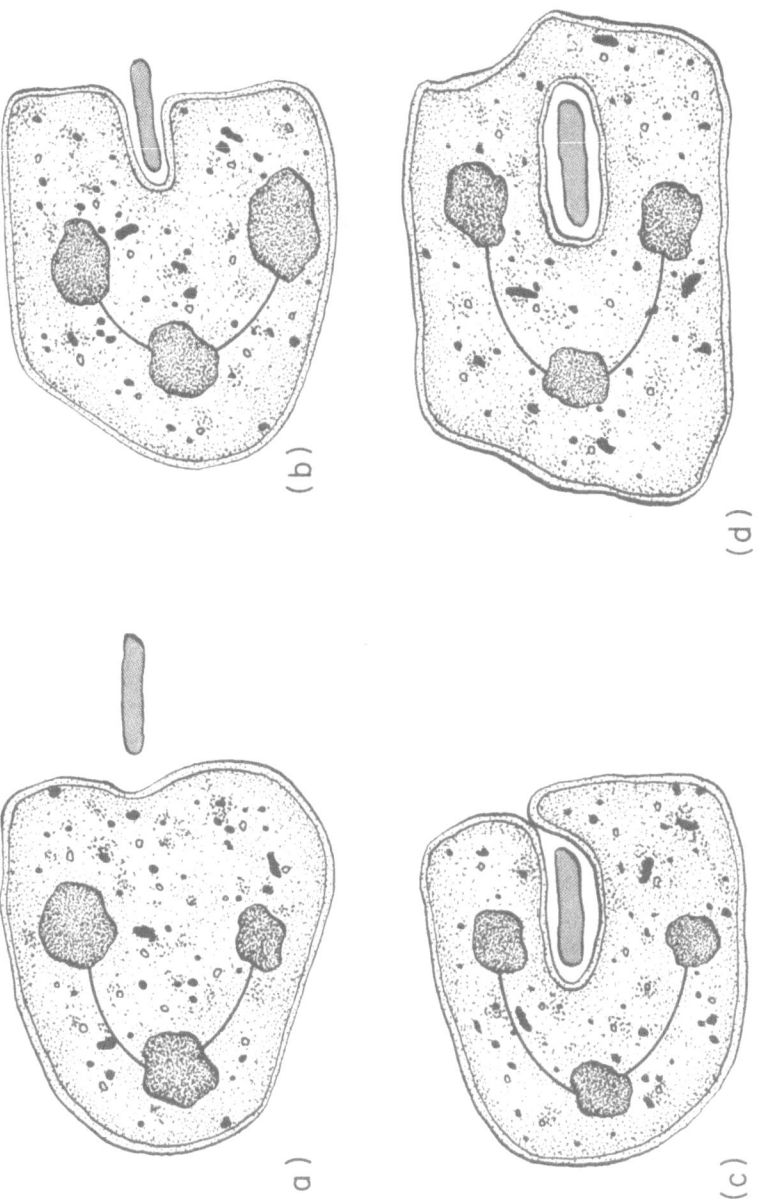

FIG. 6.1. Phagocytosis of a bacterium by a neutrophil. The inner surface of the phagocytic vesicle was the outer surface of the cell membrane.

layer of the cell membrane. The bacterium is therefore still outside the cell, in the same sense that food in the stomach is still outside the body. The phagocytic vesicle is originally connected to the cell surface by two apposed layers of cell membrane, but these soon disappear, and the vesicle with its contained bacterium is free to sink into the endoplasm of the neutrophil.

It is curious how late the significance of this mechanism was appreciated. The process of pinocytosis, or enfolding of liquid droplets by pouches of cell membrane, was described by Lewis in 1931, but throughout the 1930s and 1940s, it was vigorously denied that phagocytosis and pinocytosis had anything in common. There is no evidence that even when the true mechanism of phagocytosis was described and illustrated in electron micrographs published in 1956 by Goodman, its functional significance was appreciated. Not until 1962, when James Hirsch was trying to figure out how neutrophils killed bacteria without killing themselves in the process, was the fact that phagocytosed organisms remained extracellular integrated into a complete picture of how neutrophils go about their business.

The first person to attempt to explain how phagocytosis occurred was Ponder, who, in 1928, analyzed the problem in terms of the surface tensions between the particle and the fluid (S_1), the cell and the fluid (S_2), and the cell and the particle (S_{12}).[1] He considered an equilibrium state, in which the particle stuck to the cell surface, but was not taken up, and showed that

$$S_1 = S_{12} + S_2 \cos \Theta \qquad \text{(Fig. 6.2)}$$

Thus,

$$\cos \Theta = \frac{S_1 - S_{12}}{S_2}$$

If $\cos \Theta < 1$, then a real value of Θ exists, and the particle will indeed stick and not be ingested. If $\cos \Theta > 1$, ingestion of the particle will occur; if $\cos \Theta < -1$, the particle will not stick to the cell, and ingestion is impossible. Thus, phagocytosis is favored by anything tending to make $\cos \Theta > 1$, and inspection of the equation shows that these favorable factors are an increase in the particle–fluid tension (S_1), a decrease in the cell–particle tension (S_{12}), and a decrease in the cell–fluid tension (S_2).

This type of analysis is now unfashionable. None of the three quantities is easily measurable, and in any case, the equation really applies to the situation in which one droplet (of oil, say) enters, sticks to, or is

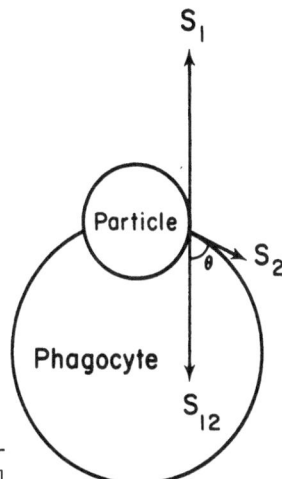

FIG. 6.2. Ponder's formulation of phagocytosis in terms of surface tension. [From Mudd *et al.*, *Physiol Rev.* **14**:210 (1934).]

rejected by another droplet (of water, say). It is by no means obvious that
the formulation is correct for a situation in which a particle is enveloped in a
piece of the cell membrane without actually entering the cytoplasm. And
yet, buried in the old literature are numberous pieces of information
strongly suggesting that surface forces and zeta potentials do have a major
influence on whether phagocytosis occurs or not. Perhaps the most interesting are the studies of Neufeld and Etinger-Tulczynska, who showed that
capsulated Type I pneumococci, which are not phagocytosed at all in a
saline medium, can be taken up in the presence of minute amounts of
trivalent cations such as Fe^{3+}, Al^{3+}, and Cr^{3+}.[2] This type of information is
of interest in two respects: It strongly suggests that the zeta potential of the
bacteria is a major factor in their resistance to phagocytosis, and it permits
one to wonder whether the "receptors" for immunoglobulin and C3b that
we will discuss later are quite as specific as is usually thought.

It is now clear that phagocytosis is not merely a passive process.
Energy is required; as mentioned, neutrophils derive most of their energy
from glycolysis, and inhibitors of this pathway such as 2-deoxyglucose
block phagocytosis. We saw earlier that the muscle system is probably
involved in phagocytosis, and if it is, ATP would be required. This may also
explain another old observation: that calcium is required for phagocytosis,
and that other cations will not substitute for it.

Nonspecific factors that strongly influence phagocytosis are the pH,
the osmotic pressure, and the temperature. Neutrophils phagocytose best

at about pH 7.3, but are not seriously interfered with until the pH falls below 6.0. Many inflammatory exudates are mildly acidic, but it seems improbable that the pH often falls below 6.0 *in vivo,* except in the urine. However, the osmotic pressure does have a profound effect on phagocytosis, and quite mild degrees of hypertonicity are measurably inhibitory. Inflammatory sites become hypertonic after injury, even when no frank tissue necrosis occurs. The maximum osmolarity after a mild burn averages 30 mosmol/liter above the normal, and is reached about 4 hr after injury.[3] The raised osmotic pressure is presumably due to enzymatic breakdown of macromolecules into their components, and is a mild version of the change seen in pus. One area of the body that is characteristically hypertonic is the renal medulla, where the osmotic pressure at the tips of the papillae may reach 1200 mosmol/liter, or 4 times the plasma osmolarity. The renal medulla is notoriously susceptible to infection, although decreased phagocytosis is only part of the explanation. Fever is a characteristic response to infection, and will be discussed in Chapter 8. In the old literature, there are many papers claiming that a rise in temperature leads to more efficient phagocytosis. Because the methodology was unsatisfactory, this idea was ridiculed by Bennett and Nicastri in 1960,[4] and has not been approached with more modern techniques. It is true that the usable range of adjustment of body temperature in man is only 3.5°C, from 37 to 40.5°C, because above 40.5°C, one starts getting near the thermal death point of the species. However, some of the papers claim significant changes with 2°C rises in temperature, and it would seem worthwhile to take another look. Also, the range of temperature adjustment in a peripheral part such as the hand may be much greater than 3.5°C.

The organism that has most often been used for studies of phagocytosis is the pneumococcus. There are several reasons for this choice. One is that until the advent of penicillin, pneumococcal pneumonia was one of the most common causes of death, and many of the people who died were in the prime of life. A more scientific reason is that the pneumococcus is a particularly simple organism. The secret of its success is its capsule, which clearly prevents phagocytosis when organism and neutrophils are incubated together in liquid media or on glass slides. Organisms that have lost their capsule by mutation or by enzymatic treatment are rapidly taken up. The pneumococcus has virtually no capacity to survive within neutrophils; if it is taken up, it is destroyed within 15 min. A patient with untreated pneumococcal pneumonia remains very ill for about 7 days; then there is a "crisis," after which rapid improvement occurs. It can be shown that antibody first appears in the serum at this time. Virulent pneumococci treated with antibody show a swelling of the capsule (the quellung phenomenon), and are readily taken up and killed by neutrophils. The accepted pathogenesis of pneumococcal pneumonia in the 1930s was that the organisms flourished until day 6 or 7, when antibody became available, whereupon they all became opsonized and were destroyed.

6.1.2. Surface Phagocytosis

W. Barry Wood performed a rather simple test to see whether this idea was true: He looked at sections of lung from people who had died early in the course of pneumococcal pneumonia to see whether phagocytosis had in fact occurred. He had no difficulty finding neutrophils that had phagocytosed pneumococci, and indeed in the older (central) parts of the pneumonic area, pneumococci were hard to find. The only portion of the lesion with numerous free pneumococci was the edema zone on the outside, where neutrophils had not yet arrived (Fig. 6.3). He therefore injected pneumococci into the footpad of a rat, and demonstrated neutrophils containing pneumococci within 30 min, both at the injection site and in the local lymph nodes. He also injected pneumococci down the rat trachea, and demonstrated phagocytosis in that site.

There was no evidence that these rats had antipneumococcal antibody; the pneumococcus does not naturally infect rodents, and the neutrophils of the animals were quite unable to phagocytose pneumococci when incubated with them in normal rat serum in tubes or on glass slides. And yet, mixtures of rat neutrophils and pneumococci showed obvious phagocytosis if they were introduced into normal rat lung and left there for 4 hr. There was something different about the lung that enabled phagocytosis to occur when it was impossible *in vitro*. Wood then went to extraordinary lengths to exclude antibody. He showed that phagocytosis occurred in lungs perfused with saline instead of blood, and even in lungs fixed in formalin, in which all the proteins would have been denatured. Finally, he realized that the crucial factor was the availability of a suitable surface. The decisive observation was that phagocytosis occurred in short lengths of rat bronchi, but not in glass tubes of the same diameter, even if they were lined with bronchial mucus. He rapidly demonstrated that phagocytosis of pneumococci by rat neutrophils could occur on almost any body surface, including

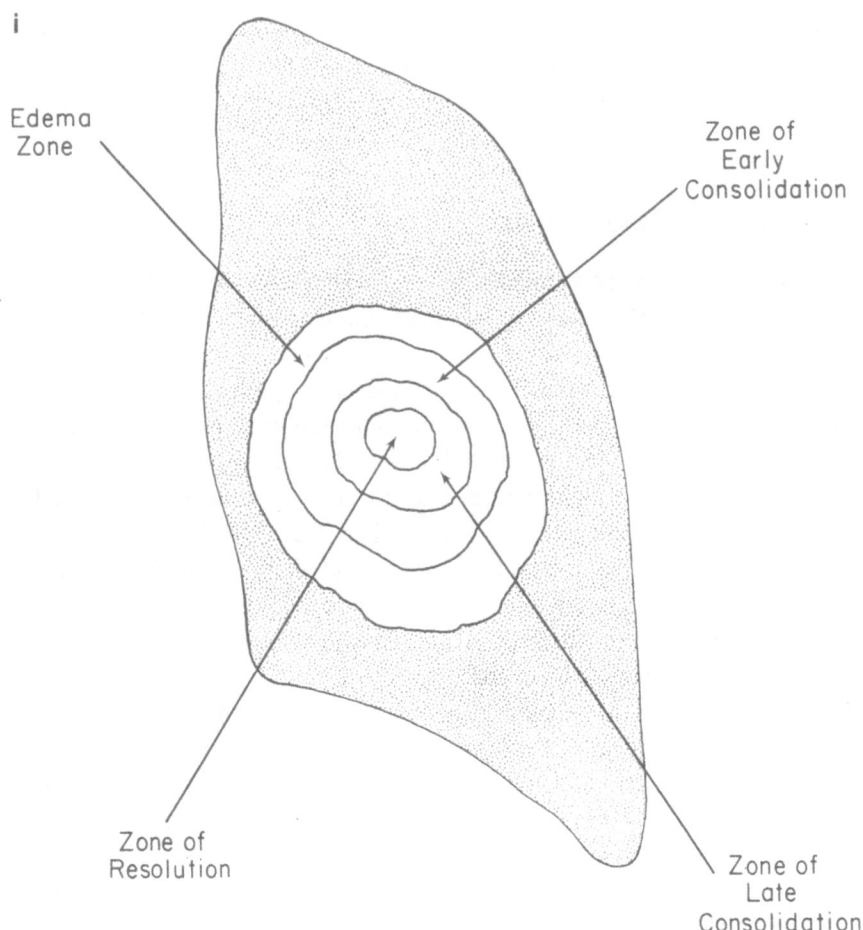

FIG. 6.3. Pneumococcal pneumonia in the rat. (1) Pneumonia starts at one focus and spreads outward. (ii) In the edema zone, neutrophils are sparse, and pneumococci are numerous. (iii) Pneumococci flourishing in a major bronchus. However, some surface phagocytosis has occurred because two of the neutrophils contain cocci. (iv) The zone of early consolidation. Neutrophils have arrived and are phagocytosing pneumococci. (v) The zone of advanced consolidation. All the bacteria are inside neutrophils. Note how the oldest, central part of the pneumonic area is almost healed, while at the outer edge, new areas of lung are still being involved by the spread of infected edema fluid from one alveolus to another. [From Wood, *J. Exp. Med.* **73**:222 (1941), and Sale and Wood, *J. Exp. Med.* **86**:248 (1947).]

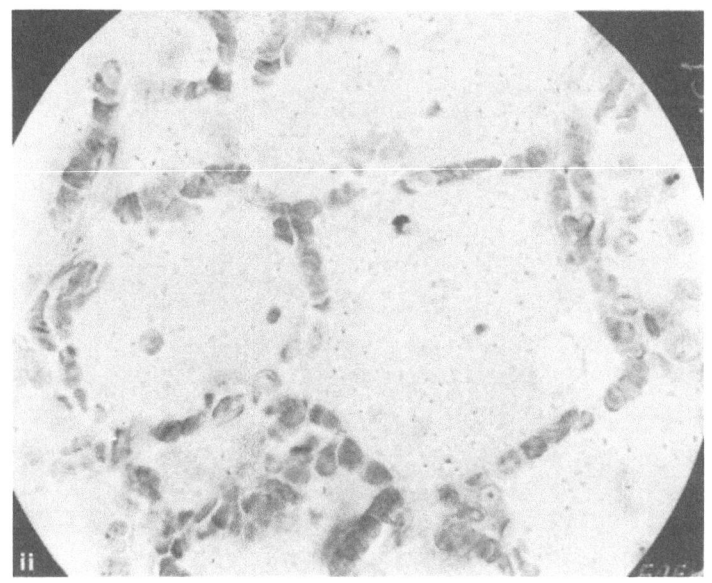

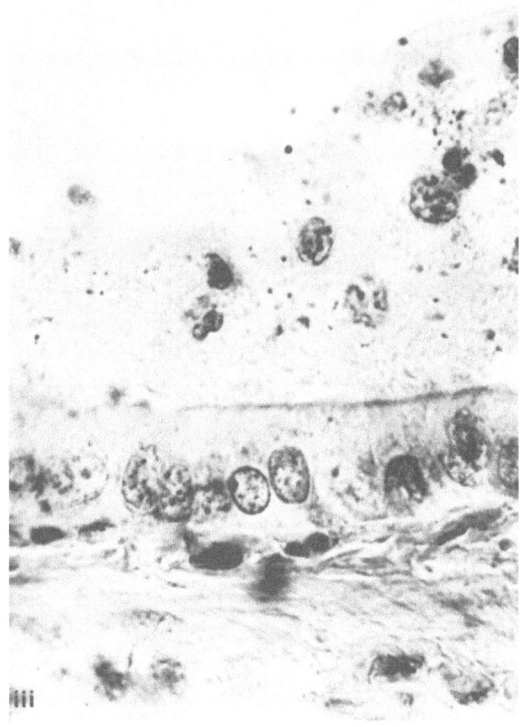

FIG. 6.3 (cont)

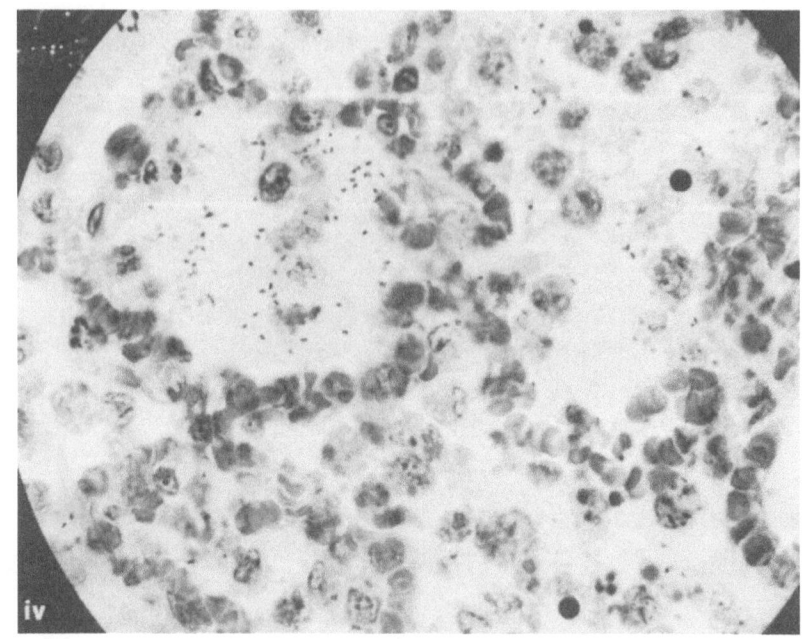

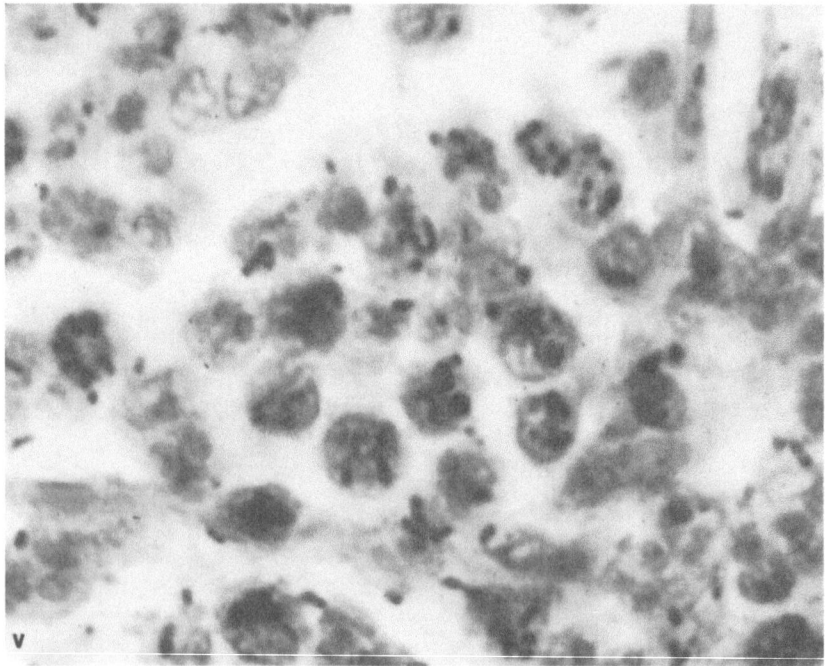

FIG. 6.3 (cont)

the trachea, esophagus, endothelium, pleura and peritoneum, muscle, and the cut surfaces of the liver, kidney, and spleen. The tissue could be boiled without affecting the result. Furthermore, a variety of structured surfaces such as fibrin clots, filter paper, fiber glass, and gelatin sponge could support phagocytosis *in vitro* when glass slides would not. He showed that if a hanging drop preparation was made using a coverslip with a small piece of filter paper attached to it, neutrophils on the paper took up pneumococci, while those in the fluid phase did not. He devised two ingenious ways of actually observing surface phagocytosis, and saw that the neutrophils trapped the organisms against a solid surface and were then able to take them up (Fig. 6.4). Finally, he showed that pneumococci taken up by surface phagocytosis were killed and digested by the cells, just as though they had been taken up after opsonization with antibody.[5]

6.1.3. The Heat-Labile Opsonin System

A second mechanism that facilitates phagocytosis in the absence of antibody is the heat-labile opsonin system, which is now known to involve the alternate pathway of complement fixation. The discovery of this mechanism had its origin in the early controversies about whether or not the opsonic activity of sera for bacteria could be destroyed by heating at 56°C. By 1910, this controversy had pretty well been resolved in favor of the view that low levels of specific antibody in normal sera were responsible for their opsonic activity, and that complement served merely to amplify the response. But reports of experiments in which anticapsular antibody seemed to be excluded persisted. Thus, Ward and Enders showed in 1933 that normal serum could promote phagocytosis of pneumococci to a limited degree, and that this opsonic activity could not be inhibited by purified capsular polysaccharide.[6] The activity could be adsorbed out by whole pneumococci, and was thought to represent antibody against cell wall components other than the capsule. On the other hand, Smith and Wood, working with a different type of pneumococcus (Type 25), also found heat-labile opsonic activity in normal serum, but showed that *E. coli* was just as effective at adsorbing out the activity as was the pneumococcus.[7] This finding made specific antibodies against pneumococcal antigens an improbable explanation for the opsonic activity. Furthermore, the opsonic activity was not adsorbed out at 0°C, even with repeated use of huge quantities of pneumococci. Antibodies combine perfectly well with antigens at 0°C; indeed, precipitin tests are always done at 4°C or below to ensure complete

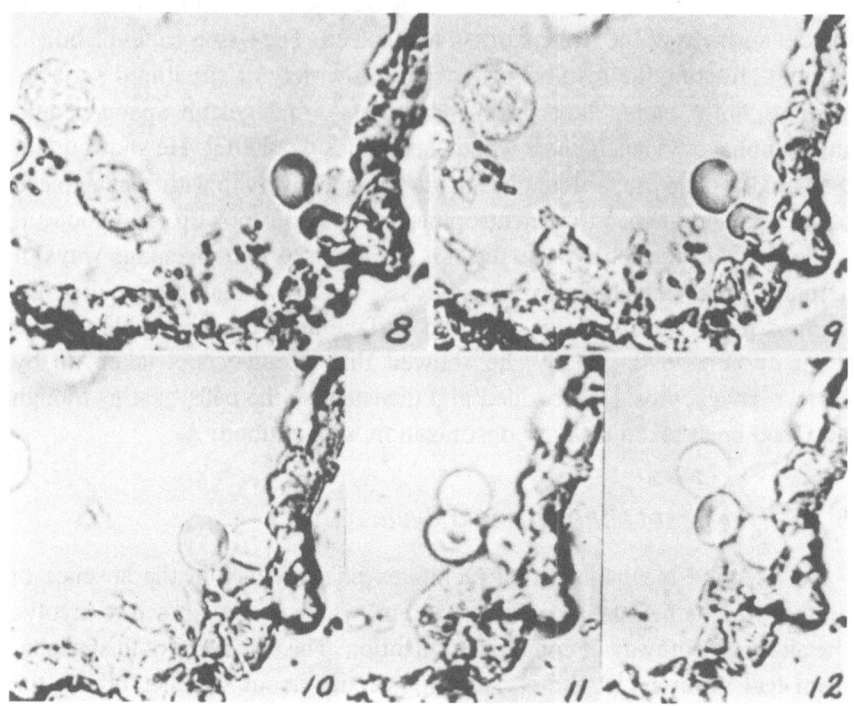

FIG. 6.4. Surface phagocytosis. A neutrophil is trapping Friedländers bacilli against the alveolar wall. [From Smith and Wood, *J. Exp. Med.* **86**:257 (1947).]

precipitation. They wondered whether complement was perhaps being fixed by some mechanism other than binding to antibody. Preliminary experiments showed that the opsonic activity of normal serum for Type 25 pneumococci had the same heat stability as complement, was absorbed out by antigen—antibody complexes, was dependent on the presence of Ca^{2+} and Mg^{2+}, and was inactivated by treatment of the serum with either zymosan or cobra venom. All these measures prevent the activity of one or more complement components.

Wood enlisted the help of H. S. Shin, who performed detailed complement component analyses on normal guinea pig serum that had opsonized pneumococci.[8] Of the C3, 80% had disappeared, with substantial amounts (20–40%) of components 5–9. However, components 1, 4, and 2 were hardly changed. It was then shown that opsonized pneumococci carried C3b on their surface (Fig. 6.5). This was done in three ways: (1) By treating them with monospecific anti-C3 antibody. This made the organisms agglutinate and produced a quellung reaction. (2) By treating them with fluorescent anti-C3 antibody. Opsonized pneumococci, but not normal pneumo-

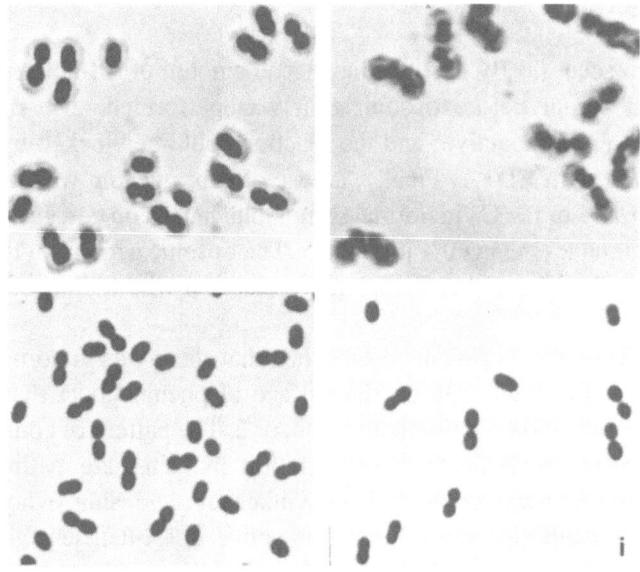

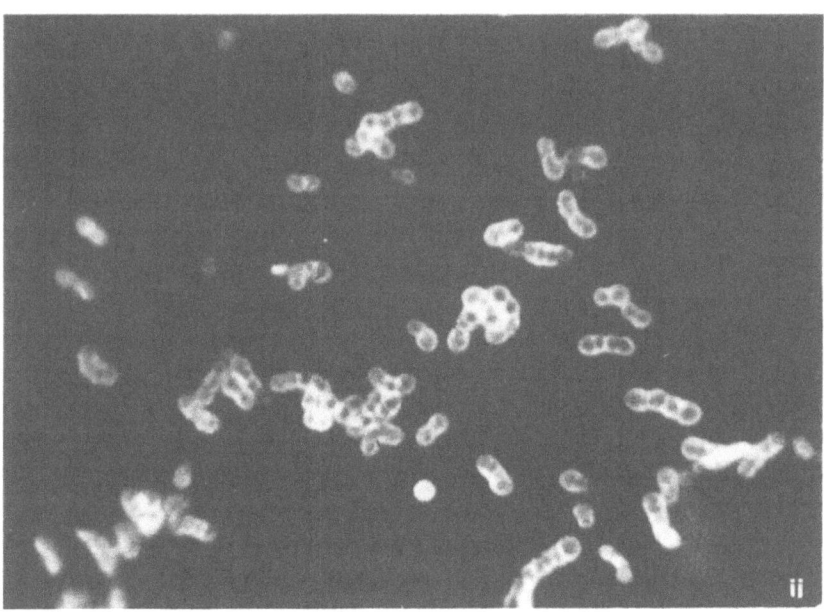

FIG. 6.5. The heat-labile opsonin system. In the upper area, on the left, are pneumococci treated with immune (above) and normal serum. The quellung phenomenon is obvious with the immune serum. On the right, at the top, are pneumococci opsonized by the HLO system and treated with antibody against C3. Again, capsular swelling is obvious. Below, right, are pneumococci treated with serum plus EDTA, which blocks the alternate pathway. They look normal. In the lower panel are pneumococci opsonized by the HLO system and treated with fluorescent antibody against C3. They are obviously fluorescent. These experiments made it clear that opsonization by the HLO system culminates in the binding of C3 to the bacterial surface. [From Shin, Smith, and Wood, *J. Exp. Med.* **130**:1229 (1969).]

cocci, fluoresced. (3) By introducing a small amount of ^{125}I-labeled C3 into the normal serum before opsonization was performed. The opsonized organisms were radioactive, and the reaction could be blocked by heating the serum, or with EDTA. Finally, a dose of cobra venom was found that inactivated 95% of the C3 in normal serum, but caused no detectable loss of C1, 4, or 2, and less than 10% loss of C5. The opsonic activity of the serum was destroyed, and could be completely restored by the addition of purified C3.

These classic experiments established that there was in normal serum a mechanism for fixing C3b on the surface of pneumococci that did not appear to require either antibody or C1, 4, or 2. The pattern of consumption of complement components suggested that the alternate pathway was involved, and this was confirmed by Winkelstein and Shin, who showed that the heat-labile opsonin system was active in C4-deficient guinea pig serum, and that it could not be blocked by anti-C2 antibody.[9] However, the later experiments spoiled the picture a little by showing that in guinea pig serum, there is in fact a role for immunoglobulin in the heat-labile opsonin system. They showed that IgG2 antibody became bound to the pneumococcal surface, and that if this antibody was removed from the serum, opsonization was much less effective, or even ineffective. Furthermore, the IgG2 antibody was probably directed against some pneumococcal antigen, because purified IgG2 anti-DNP antibody would not opsonize the pneumococcus. The specificity was not anticapsular, since it could not be absorbed out with huge quantities of capsular polysaccharide, and since they confirmed that the opsonic activity could be absorbed out with *E. coli,* the specificity is presumably directed against an antigen that is very widely distributed in bacteria. They also showed that the Fc part of the IgG2 antibody was unnecessary for opsonic activity; this finding established for certain that the complement fixation was occurring via the alternate pathway.

The conflict between the earlier results, which suggested that antibody was not involved at all, and the later work is more apparent than real, and is an example of the relativity mentioned earlier. The work was done in different species (rat *vs* guinea pig), with different strains of pneumococci, and with different concentrations of cells and bacteria. Much of the later work was done primarily by measuring C3 fixation, and phagocytic tests were done only for confirmation, or not at all. It would probably be fair to say that the alternate pathway can be initiated in the total absence of antibody, but that under natural conditions, there are always traces of antibodies directed against common bacterial components, and these anti-bodies potentiate complement fixation by the alternate pathway.

6.1.4. Opsonization Mediated by Antibodies

In the *Introduction,* it was mentioned that early workers found that the antibodies in normal serum usually required complement for their opsonic activity, whereas antibodies in the sera of highly immunized animals did not. The first glimmer of light about this situation came when Pondman separated antibodies to sheep red cells by ultracentrifugation.[10] The 19 S (IgM) antibodies were incapable of opsonizing red cells unless complement was present, whereas the 7 S (IgG) antibodies would opsonize readily by themselves. This difference, then, is the cause of the confusion. Most of the antibodies in normal serum are present in low titer and are of the IgM class. This is especially true of antibody to gram-negative organisms. IgM has no opsonic activity of its own, but is exceedingly efficient at fixing complement because only one bound molecule is required. Thus, in normal sera, the effect of added complement is large. The antibodies in highly immune sera are mostly of the IgG class, and when they are diluted enough to abolish the opsonic activity due to IgG, complement fixation is inefficient because two adjacent bound molecules are required. Thus, in highly immune sera, the effect of complement is less obvious.

Of course, provided one gets the experimental conditions right, it is easy to demonstrate that complement fixation enhances the opsonic effect of IgG antibodies. The crucial factor is to work in the presence of normal serum. Thus, Johnson and his colleagues were able to show that phagocy-tosis of the Type 2 pneumococcus opsonized with IgG antibody was not much affected by addition of complement components 1, 4, and 2, but quintupled when C3 was added.[11] Many other papers leading to the same conclusion could be quoted, and it would therefore appear that IgG anti-body is a less efficient opsonin when serum is present than when it is not. The reason is explained by the receptor studies discussed next.

6.1.5. Receptors on Neutrophil Membranes

In 1967, LoBuglio *et al.* showed that human red cells bearing IgG antibody directed against the Rhesus D determinant would adhere to human monocytes or macrophages.[12] The red cells surrounded the mono-cyte like the petals on a flower, and the technique was christened the *rosette technique.* The rosettes were quite stable to washing and mechanical disturbance, but they broke up if either IgG or its Fc portion was added to the medium. From this finding, they deduced that the free Fc portion of the antibody bound to a specific receptor on the monocyte, from which it could be displaced competitively.

Lay and Nussenzweig showed in 1968 that sheep red cells coated with IgG anti-Forssman antibody would adhere to mouse monocytes and neutrophils.[13] The binding was inhibited by free IgG. Red cells coated with IgM antibody did not adhere to phagocytic cells at all. If complement was added, one component at a time, IgM-coated cells formed no rosettes until C3 was added, but then they adhered very well (Fig. 6.6). Furthermore, this binding was not antagonized by soluble complement components. If the IgG-coated cells were allowed to fix the first four components of complement, their rosettes were no longer broken up by free IgG.

These results were interpreted as showing that phagocytic cells have two kinds of receptors, one for the Fc portion of IgG, the other for bound C3b. There are no receptors for IgM. In serum, bacteria opsonized with

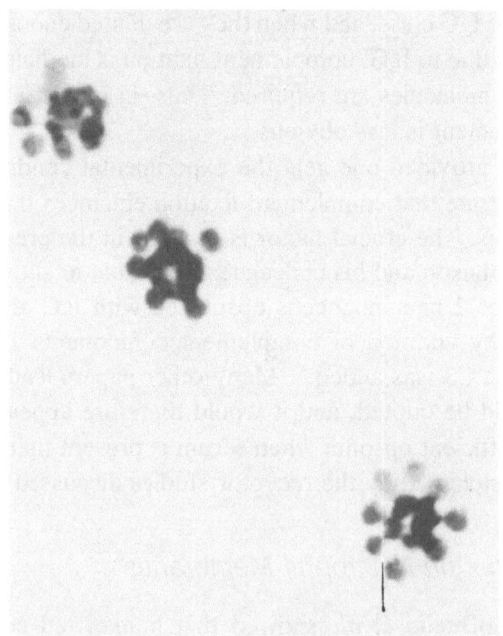

FIG. 6.6. Rosettes of erythrocytes opsonized with C1423 around neutrophils. [From Lay, W. H., and Nussenzweig, V. *J. Exp. Med.* **128:**991 (1968).[13]]

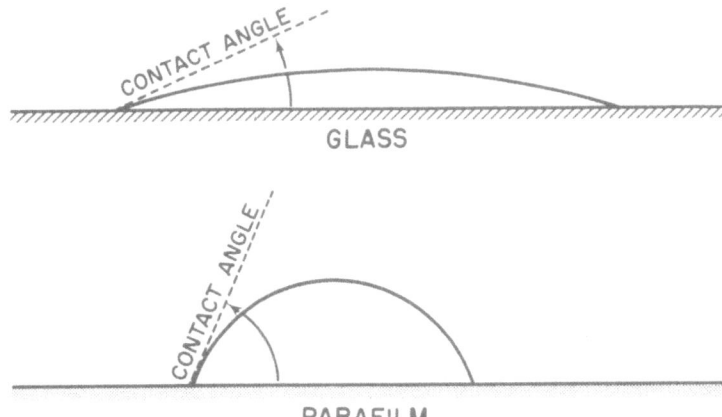

FIG. 6.7. Water drops on different surfaces. The contact angle can be measured with a goniometer, which is more usually used as an ophthalmic instrument.

IgG may not be phagocytosed because the neutrophil cannot distinguish between IgG that has fixed antigen and normal free IgG. On the other hand, C3b exposes a quite different surface from that of the normal circulating C3. There is therefore no basis for competition, and complement-mediated phagocytosis is not inhibited in the presence of serum. That there really are two separate receptors was proved by showing that the complement, but not the IgG receptors, could be destroyed by treating the cell with trypsin.

The word *receptor* conjures up the image of a membrane protein that specifically combines with, say, C3b. That this may not necessarily be the case is suggested by the work of van Oss and his colleagues.[14] They showed that the hydrophobic or hydrophilic character of a bacterial surface could be determined very simply by spreading a thick suspension of bacteria on a glass slide and allowing it to dry. A single drop of pure water is then placed on the slide, and the angle between the surface of the drop and the slide is measured. On hydrophilic surfaces (glass), the water drop tends to spread, and the angle is small. On hydrophobic surfaces (parafilm), the drop stands well up, and the angle is large (Fig. 6.7). They ranked a large number of common bacteria by this method, and found that bacteria that were easily phagocytosed had surfaces that were more hydrophobic than those of neutrophils (measured by the same technique). Capsulated bacteria had hydrophilic surfaces with respect to neutrophils, and were not easily phagocytosed. Antibody to capsulated organisms made their surfaces more hydrophobic, and simultaneously they became easier to phagocytose. The addition of C1, 4, and 2 had no effect, but when C3 was bound, both the hydrophobic character of the surface and the ease of phagocytosis increased sharply. It is therefore possible that antibody and complement aid phagocytosis because they change the character of the bacterial surface, rather than because there are specific receptor molecules for them.

In this connection, it is worth considering what an increase in hydrophobic character does to the surface tension between fluid and particle. The cause of surface tension is that the molecules at the surface of a liquid attract each other more strongly than they do those of the medium (e.g., air, glass) with which they interface. A hydrophilic surface attracts water molecules; hence, the surface tension is low. If the surface now becomes hydrophobic, the surface tension will increase. Perhaps Ponder was right after all.

However, there is some evidence suggesting that the Fc receptor of macrophages is really a specific molecule. Unkeless and Eisen studied the binding of radiolabeled immunoglobulins to macrophage layers in tissue culture.[15] Using suitable washing procedures and controls, it was possible to determine the concentration of macrophage-bound immunoglobulin (r) at several concentrations of free immunoglobulin (c). There is an established theoretical analysis (the Scatchard plot) that says that if a graph of r/c against r is linear, the affinity of the receptors for immunoglobulin is uniform. Linear plots of r/c against r were observed. Corresponding experiments with neutrophils do not appear to have been done, but it seems reasonable to suppose that a similar situation may obtain. If so, that would be evidence that a specific molecule binds IgG on neutrophil membranes.

Stossel and his colleagues have recently shown that the opsonic fragment of C3 is rather smaller than the C3b molecule that is generated during complement fixation.[16] They mixed mineral oil, a fat-soluble red dye (oil red 0), and an aqueous buffer with an emulsifying agent, either bovine serum albumin or $E.\ coli$ endotoxin. Sonication of the mixture led to the formation of an emulsion of red mineral oil droplets surrounded and stabilized by a thin film of albumin or endotoxin. Since endotoxin survives boiling, and is resistant to many enzymes and chemical agents, endotoxin-coated particles could be subjected to drastic procedures without disintegrating. Neutrophils were exposed to oil droplets opsonized with sera containing ^{125}I-labeled C3; phagocytosis could be quantitated by centrifuging and measuring the amount of red dye in the cell pellet (oil droplets themselves floated). Opsonization could be quantitated by measuring droplet-bound radioactivity.

There was an impressive correlation between ingestibility and bound radioactivity when fresh normal serum was reacted with particles. Opsonized particles retained their opsonized status when subjected to boiling in 2 M sodium chloride, 8 M urea, 2% deoxycholate, and several other dissociating agents. However, it was possible to strip off bound C3 with sodium dodecyl sulfate (SDS), and it was inferred that the binding was principally hydrophobic in nature. Electrophoresis of SDS eluates in SDS gels suggested that the opsonic fragment has a molecular weight of 140,000 and contains two chains of about 70,000 daltons each. One of these chains is present in the intact C3 molecule; the other is a cleavage product of a chain that in the intact C3 molecule is 115,000 daltons. The experiments made it clear that several proteolytic splits occurred during the reduction of the major chain from 115,000 daltons to 70,000 daltons, and that the split that forms C3b is only the first of these.

6.2. Physiological Significance of Phagocytic Mechanisms

Which of all these various phagocytic mechanisms are important in living animals or people? There is evidence suggesting that surface phagocytosis, the heat-labile opsonin system, and specific immunoglobulins may all be crucial in particular circumstances.

As regards surface phagocytosis, one might begin by remarking that it is always available, because it requires no opsonins whatever, except perhaps those that the neutrophil may bring with it. The only areas of the body in which this is not true are areas in which there are large fluid collections. Neutrophils can crawl, but they cannot swim, and urinary tract infections are among the most common illnesses. The cerebrospinal fluid is not normally exposed to infection, but meningitis resulting from implantation of small numbers of organisms during bacteremia or at surgery is almost always lethal without treatment. In mice, Wood found a strain of Group A streptococci that existed in two variants. Strain 23M produced a great deal of M protein in its capsule; strain 23G did not. Neither could be phagocytosed at all in glass tubes or on glass slides. Strain 23G was phagocytosed to a variable extent (17–37%) on filter paper, peritoneum, and other surfaces, whereas strain 23M resisted surface phagocytosis. The 23M strain was lethal for mice when one organism was injected intraperitoneally, whereas the LD_{50} for strain 23G was 1.4×10^5 organisms.[17]

There is some evidence that surface phagocytosis may play a part in clearing capsulated organisms from the bloodstream. Most bacteria injected intravenously are taken up and destroyed by the macrophages lining the sinusoids of the liver and spleen. Capsulated pneumococci, and certain other capsulated organisms such as *Klebsiella pneumoniae*, cannot be so removed unless antibody is available. Intravenous injection of these organisms causes a profound leukopenia, and microscopic examination shows that the missing neutrophils are palisaded on capillary walls, especially in the lungs. Phagocytosis of bacteria can be seen in stained sections, and it can be visualized directly in the rabbit ear chamber. The neutrophils appear to trap organisms between each other's surfaces and against the capillary walls.[18]

The heat-labile opsonin system is also available at the onset of infection, although its efficiency will be influenced by whether or not the host has traces of antibody against the organism. Actually, it may legitimately be doubted whether there is such a thing as an organism for which no antibody whatever is available: Antigens may be shared in common among the most diverse organisms; antigens of similar but not identical chemical composition will often cross-react; and, finally, if modern theories of antibody formation are anything like correct, traces of any antibody that the animal can make should be secreted in the absence of stimulation. One factor that may make traces of antibody inadequate is that the outer layer of the pneumococcal capsule is constantly becoming solubilized and diffusing away, taking with it any antibody that may have attached. Recently, the meningococcus has been shown to shed its endotoxin in the same way.

There is ample evidence of complement fixation by the alternate pathway early in bacterial infections. In 1956, when only "properdin" could be measured, Hinz showed that its level dropped to less than 10% of normal on the first day of pneumococcal pneumonia, and remained low for 6–7 days.[19] Recently, consumption of properdin and factor B has been demonstrated during gram-negative bacteremia in man.[20] Presumably, at least some of these components are being usefully employed in the opsonization of bacteria. Negative evidence that this is so is provided by the C4-deficient guinea pig and the C2-deficient human. Neither has any unusual susceptibility to infectious illness, although the classical pathway of complement fixation is completely inoperative. Positive evidence that defects of the alternate pathway lead to clinically important opsonic defects is more difficult to come by, because patients with such defects usually have other things the matter with them. Thus, children with sickle cell anemia certainly have an alternate pathway defect,[21] but they also have chronic intravascular hemolysis, which is known to depress splenic clearance of microorganisms, and they have anoxic and necrotic areas in many organs because of vascular obstruction. However, the man referred to earlier who lacked a regulator protein and turned over his alternate pathway all the time was discovered because of recurrent bacterial infections.[22]

The best-known immunoglobulin deficiency is the sex-linked variety described by Bruton, in which all serum immunoglobulins are absent or almost absent. These boys develop recurrent pyogenic infections beginning some time after 6 months of age, when the gamma globulin they received transplacentally from their mothers has been catabolized. The most common infecting organisms are pneumococci, streptococci, staphylococci, meningococci, and other capsulated organisms that are difficult to phagocytose unless antibody is available. Limited deficiencies in which only IgG is depressed are known, and are associated with the same symptoms. Even if IgM levels are raised, they cannot compensate for a deficiency in IgG, perhaps because the very high molecular weight of IgM (1 million daltons) ensures that normal capillaries are almost totally impermeable to it, and tissue levels are therefore inadequate.

However, selective IgM deficiency is also associated with greatly increased susceptibility to infectious disease, especially septicemia with capsulated organisms. In the bloodstream, there is no problem about access of IgM to bacteria, and here its superior complement-fixing ability has full play. A beautiful demonstration of this ability was given in mice by Hill and Robbins.[23] They immunized a horse against the Type I pneumococcus, and precipitated the antipneumococcal immunoglobulins with purified Type 1 polysaccharide. After the precipitates were washed, they were dissociated at pH 3.5, and the immunoglobulins were separated into IgM, IgA, and IgG fractions. They thus prepared antibodies that were directed only against the pneumococcus and the class of which was known. One hundred pneumococci were opsonized *in vitro* with known weights of the different antibodies, and were then injected into the peritoneal cavity of mice. The infection was invariably lethal unless the pneumococci were adequately opsonized; the weight of IgG required to enable 50% of the animals to survive was about 1 μg, whereas IgM was effective at 0.00001 μg.

It was remarked above that the neutrophil might perhaps bring opsonins with it. Two examples of this happening are known: The IgG receptors on neutrophils carry a random sample of whatever immunoglobulins are present in the serum, and these immunoglobulins will be translated with the cell into an inflammatory site. It has been shown that opsonizing antibodies for staphylococci and *E. coli* are so carried. The other opsonin carried on neutrophil surfaces is tuftsin, which is a tetrapeptide made in the spleen that circulates attached to IgG molecules by noncovalent bonds. When the IgG is adsorbed to neutrophils, tuftsin is transferred to the cell surface. Its structure has been determined and is thr–lys–pro–arg. It can be shown that tuftsin aids in the phagocytosis of staphylococci, and its discoverer suggested that tuftsin deficiency was one reason for the increased susceptibility of splenectomized patients to septicemia.[24]

The vast majority of bacteria are rapidly killed when they are phagocytosed by neutrophils. For them, the crucial event that determines their survival or destruction is phagocytosis. Organisms that have no special mechanism enabling them to evade phagocytosis are not pathogenic, except perhaps when they are injected in overwhelming numbers. Pathogenic organisms that can resist phagocytosis are known as *extracellular parasites*. They usually cause acute disease that either kills the host rapidly or terminates when antibody directed against the surface layers becomes available. Immunity to such infections is usually permanent, and second attacks of diseases like pneumococcal pneumonia or streptococcal sore throat are almost always due to a different strain of the organism. The situation with gram-negative rods has been complicated because many of them are not obviously capsulated, and all have endotoxin in their walls that was thought to contribute to their pathogenic effects. However, evidence is now accumulating that organisms such as *E. coli* and *Pseudomonas aeruginosa* are opsonized by antibody in just the same way as gram-positive cocci, and that they have little or no capacity for intracellular survival.[25] Indeed, immunization against *Pseudomonas* is currently being successfully used to prevent infections in burned patients who otherwise would be very susceptible. This new information allows one to take a very simple view of virtually all bacterial diseases. It is true that pyogenic bacteria can give rise to chronic and disabling illnesses such as intra-abdominal abscesses and infections of bones or the endocardium. In these cases, the explanation is invariably that some local factor has prevented adequate access of neutrophils to the organisms, and this will be discussed further in Chapter 8.

The only common organism that is totally unaffected by phagocytosis by neutrophils is the tubercle bacillus. Neutrophils that have the temerity to take it up are rapidly lysed, and the tubercle bacillus is released unharmed.[26] Certain other bacteria can resist the neutrophil in varying degrees—ranging from brucellae, which are almost totally resistant, to

Staphylococcus aureus, of which a tiny fraction, about 1% of the total organisms, can survive ingestion. Infections such as tuberculosis and brucellosis must be dealt with by monocytes and macrophages.

6.3. Summary

Phagocytosis is the process whereby bacteria and other small particles are taken into the cytoplasm of neutrophils. Many bacteria can be phagocytosed by neutrophils suspended in saline media contained in glass tubes, providing that pH, ionic strength, calcium concentration, and temperature are controlled at physiological values. However, most pathogenic bacteria have outer layers that interfere with phagocytosis. Such organisms can be taken up if a suitable surface is provided against which they can be trapped by neutrophils—"surface phagocytosis." If serum is present in the medium, most bacteria can fix complement by the alternate pathway, and bacteria coated with C3b in this way can more easily be taken up—the "heat-labile opsonin system." Sera containing specific antibacterial antibodies greatly potentiate phagocytosis.

Neutrophil membranes contain receptors that bind to IgG, which is therefore capable of acting as an opsonin in its own right. There are no receptors for IgM, but it fixes complement very efficiently. Since neutrophils also have membrane receptors for C3b, IgM is a good opsonin *in vivo.* It seems probable that under natural conditions, IgG-mediated opsonization also requires complement fixation. The nature of the neutrophil receptors for IgG and C3b is quite unknown, and it is not yet clear whether they recognize specific molecules or merely respond to the general character of the surface presented.

7

Degranulation and Intracellular Killing of Bacteria

7.1. Historical Aspects

Metchnikoff knew that neutrophils possessed "ferments" capable of digesting gelatin and other proteins, and that phagocytosed grains of litmus sometimes turned red. He knew that organisms taken up by neutrophils were enclosed in vacuoles and not admitted to the cytoplasm proper, and that in the vacuoles they were slowly digested. He said:

> We are at present ignorant of the precise manner in which this digestive and other destructive action is accomplished, and do not even know whether the substance which kills the microbes is a ferment or not.

In 1894, Kanthack and Hardy inserted bacteria contained in tubes or chambers into the peritoneal cavity of rabbits or under the skin.[1] Granular leukocytes accumulated, and the eosinophil granules were big enough to see clearly:

> The coarsely granular oxyphile cells were seen to apply themselves to a chain of bacilli, and to extend along it. The granules then travelled, usually in groups, to those portions of the cell in immediate contact with the bacilli, and there they were seen to diminish in size to mere points, and ultimately to disappear. The rate of loss of granular substance is very rapid . . . for an appreciable diminution may be observed in a quarter of an hour.

Kanthack and Hardy knew that antibacterial substances could be extracted from lymph nodes, and suggested that leukocytes killed bacteria by discharging onto them analogous substances from their granules.

Here was a virtually complete description of bacterial killing in neutrophils, but the observations were submitted to the great physiologist C. S. Sherrington, who could not confirm them, and they were forgotten.

Other early workers attempted to explain bacterial killing by the low pH ($\sim$ 5) that was thought to exist in neutrophil cytoplasm. Alexander Fleming discovered a basic protein, lysozyme, which hydrolyzed the cell walls of some bacteria. However, most of the susceptible bacteria were nonpathogenic, and some organisms that the neutrophil was known to kill were resistant to lysozyme. Various substances from normal tissues were found to kill bacteria, but since they were released only following disruption of cells, it seemed unlikely that they could be of physiological importance.

7.2. Phagocytin

The first real progress toward a solution was made by Hirsch in 1956.[2] He showed that neutrophils collected from peritoneal exudates in the rabbit would kill a variety of bacteria, both gram-positive and gram-negative, and that when the cells were disrupted by freezing and thawing, the bacteria were still killed. This effect survived dilution in buffer in pH 7.4, but was destroyed by boiling; thus, it was not due to lactic acid. As none of the bacteria were susceptible to lysozyme, the bactericidal effect could not be attributed to that. Hirsch christened the unknown principle *phagocytin*, and set about discovering more about it.

He first showed that the substance was found only in neutrophils. This finding was important because it differentiated phagocytin from the antibacterial substances such as histones, which could be extracted from any tissue by drastic procedures. He also established that phagocytin was best extracted from neutrophils at pH 4–5, that it killed a variety of organisms without lysing them, and that it worked best at a pH of about 5. It was so labile that all attempts at purification led to loss of activity.

Cohn and Hirsch then attempted to determine whether phagocytin was associated with a particular subcellular fraction.[3] They disrupted neutrophils in 0.34 M sucrose and isolated the granules by differential centrifugation. They proved to be easily lysed by acid (pH 5), but not by detergents. They contained more than 75% of the total phagocytin of the cells, and in addition, they contained an array of acid hydrolases such as acid phosphatase, RNAse, DNAse, nucleotidases, and β-glucuronidase. Cohn and Hirsch therefore suggested that the granules were lysosomes.

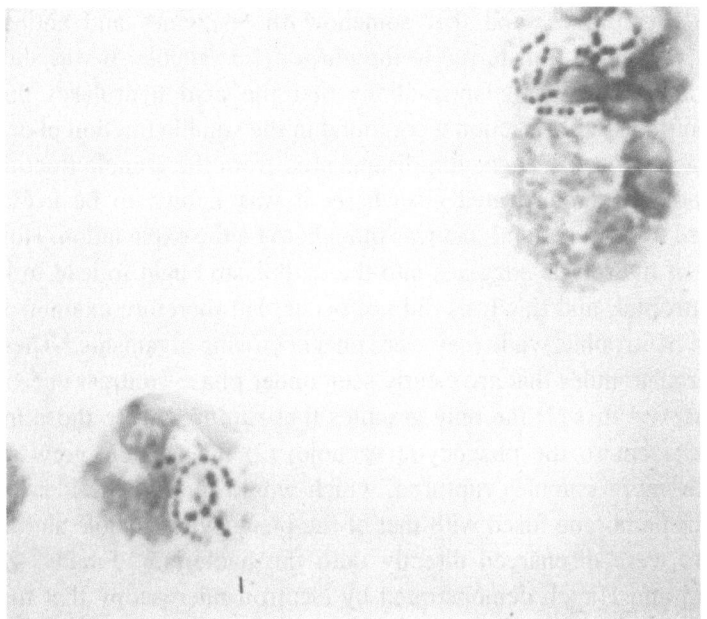

FIG. 7.1. Degranulation of rabbit neutrophils that have phagocytosed streptococci. [From Hirsch, J. G., and Cohn, Z. A., *J. Exp. Med.* **112**:1005 (1960).[4]]

7.3. Degranulation

The granules were membrane-bound, and until their membranes were ruptured, no enzymatic or bactericidal activity appeared. If the contained substances were to be of use in killing bacteria, a method had to be found for freeing the latent activities. Hirsch and Cohn therefore allowed neutrophils to phagocytose bacteria, and examined them microscopically to see whether any change in the granules had occurred.[4] They were rewarded for a brilliant piece of deductive reasoning by the rediscovery of the degranulation phenomenon (Fig. 7.1). They showed that loss of granules occurred following phagocytosis of almost any organism, and that its extent varied with the number ingested. Neutrophils that had not taken up organisms retained their granules, those with one or two were partially degranulated, those with several had lost all granules. If a cell was partially degranulated, the remaining granules looked normal. They showed that granular enzymes did not appear in the medium; thus, granules were somehow being used within the cell.

Hirsch at first thought it likely that the lactic acid produced by increased glycolysis lowered the pH of the cytoplasm, leading to rupture of granule membranes, and that somehow the enzymes and antibacterial protein were then transferred to the phagocytic vacuole. It was shown by examination of subcellular fractions that the acid hydrolases normally found in the granule fraction were found in the soluble fraction of cells that had phagocytosed. Phagocytin disappeared from the granule fraction, and could not be demonstrated elsewhere; it was known to be irreversibly adsorbed to bacteria, and that was thought to be the explanation. However, release of hydrolytic enzymes into the cytoplasm ought to lead to lysis of the neutrophil, and this lysis did not occur. He therefore examined living chicken neutrophils while they were phagocytosing organisms.[5] These cells have large granules that are clearly seen under phase-contrast microscopy. He observed that (1) the only granules that ruptured were those immediately adjacent to the phagocytic vacuole; (2) the vacuole grew steadily larger as more granules ruptured, which would fit with the idea that the granular membrane fused with that of the phagocytic vacuole and that the contents were discharged directly onto the bacterium. Finally, Zucker-Franklin and Hirsch demonstrated by electron microscopy that fusion of the membranes of the granules and phagocytic vacuole did in fact occur, and that the bacteria became covered with granular contents[6] (Fig. 7.2).

This beautiful mechanism ensures that bacteria are killed and digested without exposing the cell to its own destructive enzymes. Hirsch's morphological observations have been confirmed biochemically by many workers. Perhaps the neatest demonstration was by Stossel and his co-workers, who allowed cells to phagocytose oil droplets enclosed in a layer of bovine serum albumin.[7] The oil droplets had a low density, so if the neutrophils were gently lysed after phagocytosis, the phagocytic vesicles would float when put on a sucrose gradient in the ultracentrifuge. The granules and other cell organelles moved down the gradient, and it was possible to show transfer of various enzymes from the specific and azurophil granule bands into the phagocytic vesicles. Another way of showing the same thing is to use histochemical techniques; peroxidase is particularly convenient, because it can be made to yield a densely electron-opaque reaction product.

7.3.1. Specific Degranulation

Bainton found evidence that the specific granules fused with the phagocytic vesicle first, the process starting at about 30 sec after ingestion.[8] Azurophil granules did not begin to discharge their contents until 3 min, and usually only into the larger vesicles. This finding raised the possibility that

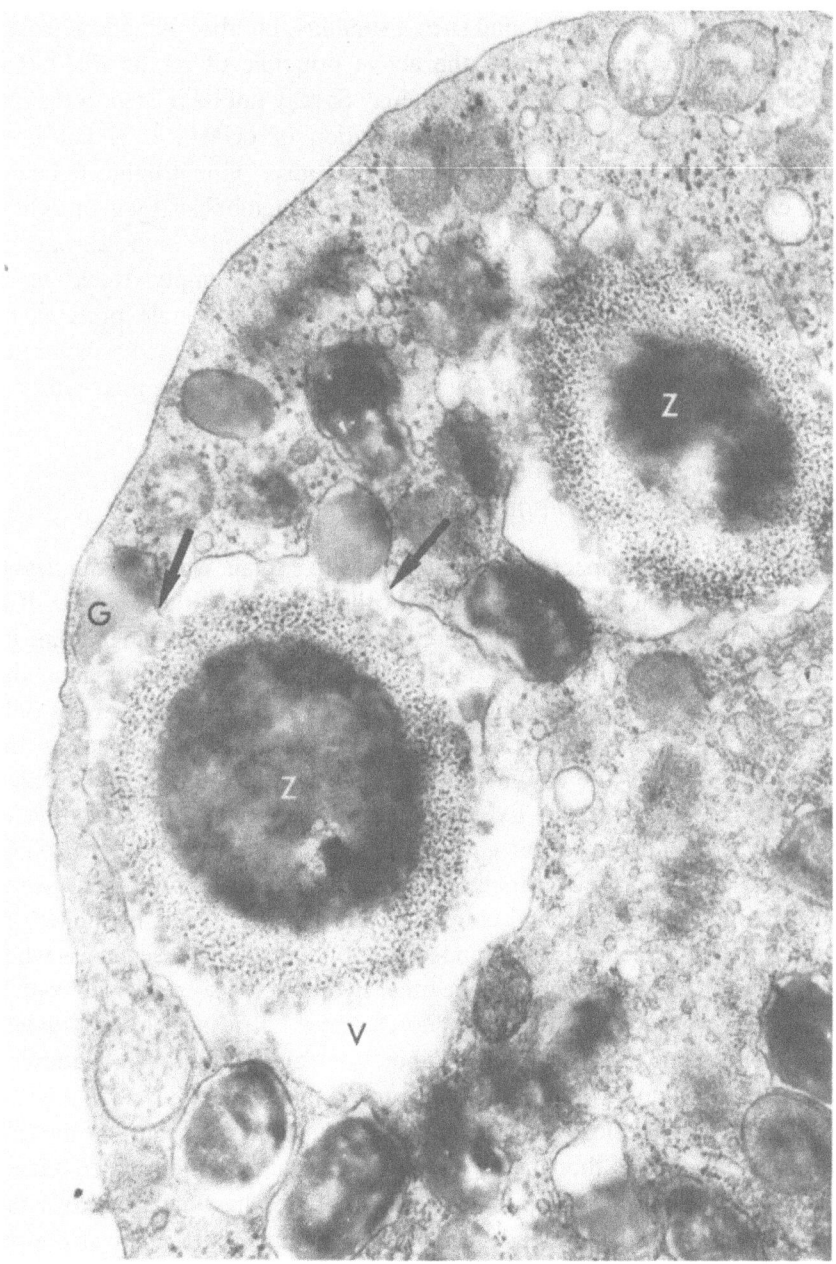

FIG. 7.2. Electron micrograph of degranulation following phagocytosis of zymosan. Fusion of the granular and phagocytic vesicle membranes is clearly shown. [From Zucker-Franklin, D., and Hirsch, J. G., *J. Exp. Med.* **120:**569 (1964).[6]]

some stimuli might cause degranulation of only one type of granule. Estensen and co-workers found such a stimulus, phorbol myristic acetate.[9] This compound is an irritant, the active principle of croton oil. It has various effects on neutrophils, which may or may not be related to the fact that it raises the intracellular concentration of cGMP. It is not itself chemotactic, but markedly enhances the responses of neutrophils to bacterial chemotactic factors; it stimulates oxidative metabolism by neutrophils; and it causes degranulation of the specific granules only, in the absence of intracellular particles. The affected cells develop large empty vesicles in the cytoplasm that can be shown to contain specific granule proteins by histochemical methods. It is of some interest that vacuolated polymorphs are found in the blood during bacteremia, and perhaps the mechanism is similar.

7.3.2. Possible Membrane-Fusion Mechanisms

One puzzling aspect of degranulation is to explain why the granules do not fuse with the plasma membrane of the cell, or with each other. It is possible to suppose that granules are kept away from the cell membrane by the microfilament meshwork, but this cannot be the whole explanation, because cells treated with cytochalasin B degranulate to the exterior only when exposed to particles. There must be some kind of change in the internal surface of the cell membrane when it comes into contact with a phagocytoseable particle. Evidence that changes in the organization of neutrophil membranes occur during phagocytosis was provided by Romeo et al., using a fluorescent probe.[10] 1-Anilinonaphthalene-8-sulfonate (ANS) absorbs light at 379 nm and emits it at 475 nm. If ANS is in solution in water, its fluorescence is only modest; a pronounced increase occurs when it is transferred to benzene or some other hydrophobic solvent. Neutrophils incubated with ANS show some fluorescence, but if particles are added, the fluorescence increases sharply (about fourfold) within 2 sec. Naturally, one does not know whether the conformational change is occurring in the cell membrane or the granule membranes, but 2 sec is so short a time that one would not have thought any granule membranes could have contacted the particles. Furthermore, once the fluorescence has increased over the first 2 sec, it remains steady for at least 5 min, although ingestion of particles and degranulation must be going on.

Hirsch has evidence that the membranes of rabbit specific granules are very different from those of the azurophil granules.[11] He isolated pure granule populations by differential centrifugation, and then disrupted them by freezing and thawing. The purified membranes differed in their choles-terol-to-phospholipid ratios (azurophil, 0.49; specific, 0.36). Furthermore, when the membrane proteins were separated by SDS electrophoresis, it was shown that each membrane had 10–15 components, and that scarcely any of these components were held in common. Whether these major differences in granule membrane composition have anything to do with the early fusion of specific granules is not known.

The whole question of why one membrane fuses with another is under very active investigation at present, because it is an essential feature of vital cell functions such as the fertilization of ova and mitosis. Lucy has discov-ered a number of simple lipids that promote fusion of one cell with another.[12] One is lysolecithin, which causes many different types of cells to form multinucleated giant cells. Such giant cells are very unstable, and soon break up completely. However, Lucy pointed out that localized and transient production of lysolecithin by enzymes at the cell surface might promote fusion without threatening the integrity of the cell as a whole. Subsequently, he showed that unsaturated fatty acids and medium-chain (C_{10}–C_{14}) saturated fatty acids could also induce membrane fusion. These observations have been synthesized into the working hypothesis that sub-stances promoting cell fusion do so by causing a change in the cell mem-brane lipids from the bilayer to the globular micelle form.[13] One supposes that similar membrane alterations underlie the degranulation of neutrophils (Fig. 7.3).

7.4. Intracellular Killing of Bacteria

Phagocytin was envisioned as an antibacterial substance that could be extracted from cells, but was in no way dependent on them for its function. Evidence that important bactericidal mechanisms were dependent on the oxidative metabolism of the neutrophil developed from two independent directions.

7.4.1 Oxygen and Bacterial Killing

In the first place, a series of workers beginning with Selvaraj and Sbarra in 1966 showed that although neutrophils could phagocytose organ-isms perfectly well in the absence of oxygen, some bacteria were killed either very poorly or not at all.[14] A recent study by Mandell was typical, in

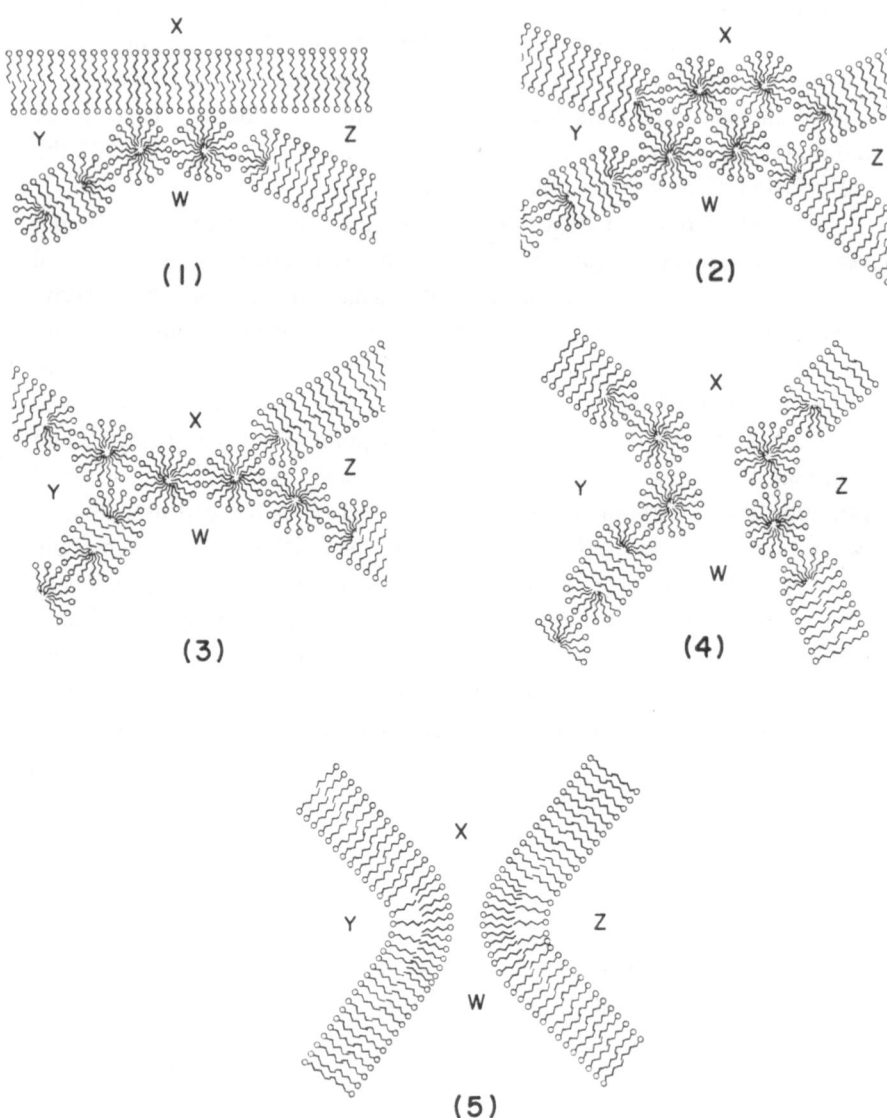

FIG. 7.3. A possible scheme for membrane fusion. [From Lucy, J. A., *Nature* **227**:815 (1970).[13]]

that staphylococci, *Serratia marcescens,* and various enterobacteria were found to survive well in neutrophils held under anerobic conditions.[15] Representatives of several other major bacterial familes were killed normally, including *Staphylococcus epidermidis, Streptococcus faecalis, Streptococcus viridans, Pseudomonas aeruginosa,* peptococci, peptostreptococci, *Clostridium perfringens,* and *Bacteroides fragilis.*

7.4.2. Myeloperoxidase

The second line of evidence developed out of some work on the etiology of dental caries, performed by Seymour Klebanoff. It was known that germ-free rats did not develop caries, whatever diet they were fed. When normal rats were fed a cariogenic (high-sucrose) diet, there were pronounced individual variations in how much caries developed. It seemed possible that antibacterial substances in saliva altered the mouth flora and were responsible for these variations.

It was soon found that centrifuged saliva contained something that prevented lactobacilli from growing. Dialysis of saliva abolished the activity, and combining the dialyzed protein with the dialyzate restored it. It was then shown that the dialyzable cofactor was the thiocyanate ion, CNS^-, which is present in concentrations of up to 27 mg/100ml in normal saliva. The nondialyzable portion was destroyed by heating, and was thought to be a protein. Peroxidase was known to be one of the proteins present in saliva, and was known to mediate various oxidative processes with the help of hydrogen peroxide. Catalase destroys hydrogen peroxide, and Klebanoff found that adding catalase to saliva abolished its bacteriostatic power. Peroxidase was known to occur also in milk and in neutrophils; even better, methods for purifying the enzyme from these sources were available. It was now shown that purified peroxidase, hydrogen peroxide, and thiocyanate could prevent bacterial growth, and the activity in saliva was completely explained.[16] Klebanoff was fortunate in that the organism he used for testing the killing power of saliva was a lactobacillus, which was catalase-negative and thus produced its own hydrogen peroxide. Had he used a catalase-positive organism such as *Escherichia coli,* exogenous hydrogen peroxide would have been necessary, and two factors would have been removed by dialysis instead of one.

Because thiocyanate is not found in appreciable quantities in serum or most cells, Klebanoff investigated the efficiency of other ions in this

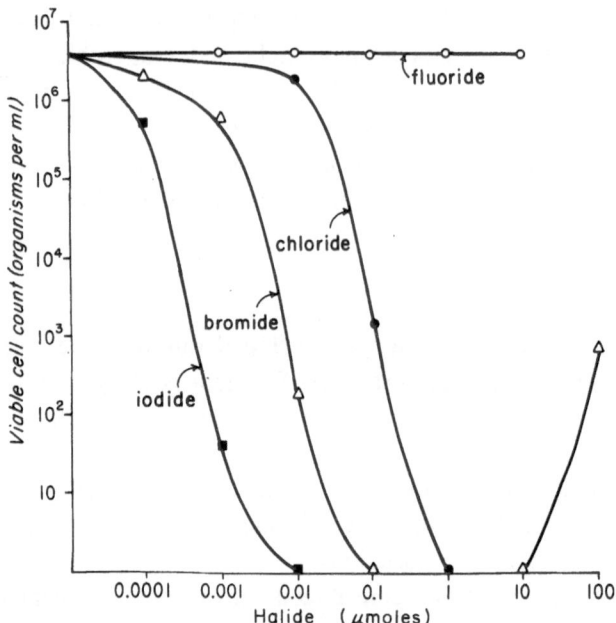

FIG. 7.4. Killing of *Escherichia coli* by myeloperoxidase, hydrogen peroxide, and various amounts of halides. The initial number of organisms was 5×10^6, and the mixtures were incubated for 30 min before the surviving bacteria were counted. Note that the chloride concentration required to completely kill this inoculum is about 1 meq/liter, or one-hundredth the amount in normal serum. [From Klebanoff, S. J., *J. Bacteriol.* **95**:2131 (1968).[17]]

system. He found that iodide, bromide, and chloride would all serve as the anion; furthermore, when halides were used, the bacteria were not merely prevented from growing, but were killed outright (Fig. 7.4). The efficiency of the system was astounding: A million *E. coli* could be killed in half an hour with only a few micrograms of peroxidase. Iodide was the most effective halide; chloride was about 100 times less efficient.[17]

Hydrogen peroxide and iodine are bactericidal in their own right, and are commonly used as disinfectants. However, the concentrations in Klebanoff's experiments were four orders of magnitude below the concentrations required for bacterial killing in the absence of peroxidase. Furthermore, it was shown that the bacteria, peroxidase, hydrogen peroxide, and iodide all had to be present in the mixture together; if the bacteria were added 10 min after the other three were mixed, no killing occurred. This finding suggested that I_2 was not the bactericidal agent, and that perhaps nascent iodine might be involved. This suspicion was confirmed by showing that $^{125}I^-$ was incorporated into tyrosine residues in the bacterial cell wall.

Myeloperoxidase occurs in the azurophil granules of neutrophils, and is delivered directly into the phagocytic vesicle when degranulation occurs. Chloride is present in the cell sap in concentrations about 100 times as great as those required to kill bacteria in the *in vitro* system. Iodide is present in neutrophils in concentrations higher than those in serum; whether they are high enough to mediate bacterial killing is uncertain. Klebanoff showed that intact neutrophils could deiodinate thyroid hormones and incorporate the iodine into bacterial cell walls, so perhaps iodide itself would not be necessary. Hydrogen peroxide is generated in neutrophils by the burst of oxidative metabolism that accompanies phagocytosis, and the quantities generated are many times those required to kill bacteria in the presence of peroxidase. Just how much hydrogen peroxide is generated is difficult to say, because it can be consumed by several intracellular pathways, and one can measure only what is left over. So it seemed probable that myeloperoxidase was an important bactericidal mechanism in living neutrophils.[18]

(a) Chronic Granulomatous Disease. Chronic granulomatous disease (CGD) is a congenital disorder in which children are afflicted with recurrent bacterial infections leading to death at an early age. The organisms responsible for the infections are staphylococci and gram-negative rods, and there is no unusual incidence of infection with pneumococci or streptococci. In 1967, Holmes and Quie found that the neutrophils of these children were unable to kill staphylococci. In the same year, it was discovered that the neutrophils of patients with CGD did not show a burst of oxygen uptake when they phagocytosed organisms. This finding suggested to Kebanoff that perhaps the failure to kill staphylococci was related to the failure to generate hydrogen peroxide during phagocytosis.

Klebanoff and White therefore obtained neutrophils from patients with CGD and incubated them with $^{125}I^-$ and *Serratia marcescens*.[19] This microorganism is a catalase-positive, gram-negative rod that is frequently responsible for infections in patients with CGD. The cells took up the organisms, but autoradiographs showed that there was no accumulation of iodine in the cells. Normal neutrophils took up the organisms, and heavy radioactive labeling of the bacteria was demonstrated both by autoradiography and by breaking up the cells and isolating the organisms (Fig. 7.5). This

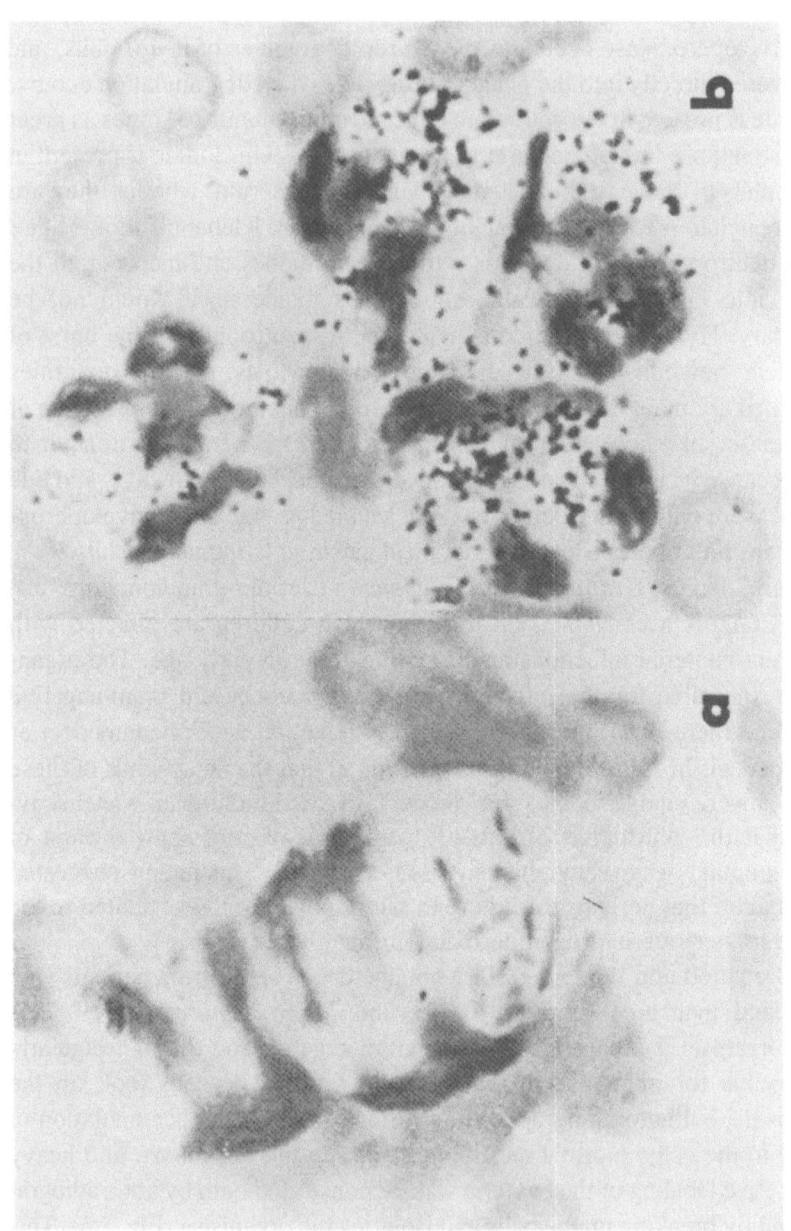

FIG. 7.5. Iodination of *Serratia marcescens* by normal neutrophils (right), but not by CGD neutrophils (left). [From Klebanoff, S. J., and White, L. R., *N. Engl. J. Med.* **280**:460 (1969).[19]]

was clear evidence that the myeloperoxidase bactericidal mechanism was defective in CGD neutrophils. CGD exists in several genetic variants, but sex-linked recessive inheritance is the most common. The mothers of these boys are clinically normal, but they are obligate carriers of the CGD abnormality. Since one X chromosome is inactive in adult females, and the inactivation is random, it might be expected that they would have two populations of neutrophils, one that iodinated bacteria and another that did not. Examination of neutrophils from the mothers of boys with CGD showed that this expectation was fulfilled[19] (Fig. 7.6).

It was also shown that catalase-negative organisms such as pneumo-cocci, streptococci, and lactobacilli produced enough hydrogen peroxide by their own metabolism to enable CGD neutrophils to kill them. Thus, the reason the children were predominantly infected by particular species of bacteria became apparent. It should be pointed out that many organisms, such as meningococci and *Hemophilus influenzae,* are catalase-positive, and yet do not cause trouble in patients with CGD. They are presumably susceptible to one of the other bactericidal mechanisms in neutrophils; only those catalase-positive organisms that cannot be killed except by the oxidative mechanisms will be important pathogens in these children.

(b) Oxidative Metabolism in Neutrophils. It would be expected that some specific enzyme concerned with hydrogen peroxide generation was defective or missing in CGD neutrophils, and this expectation necessitates a further discussion of the burst of oxidative metabolism that accompanies phagocytosis.

When neutrophils take up organisms, there follows a series of related changes: increased oxygen consumption; increased hexose monophos-phate shunt activity; increased oxidation of formate; and generation of hydrogen peroxide, superoxide, and a number of other highly reactive compounds. None of these changes occurs in the neutrophils of children with CGD. The increased oxygen consumption is not suppressed by cya-nide, which is fairly good evidence that it is not being mediated by cytochromes. It appears to be due to the activity of oxidases, enzymes that are usually flavoproteins and can couple the oxidation of a suitable sub-strate directly to molecular oxygen. The most likely substrates in neutro-phils are NADH and NADPH.

The simplest system for generating hydrogen peroxide in neutrophils would be a direct oxidation of NADPH. The first two reactions of the hexose monophosphate shunt are obligately coupled to the reduction of

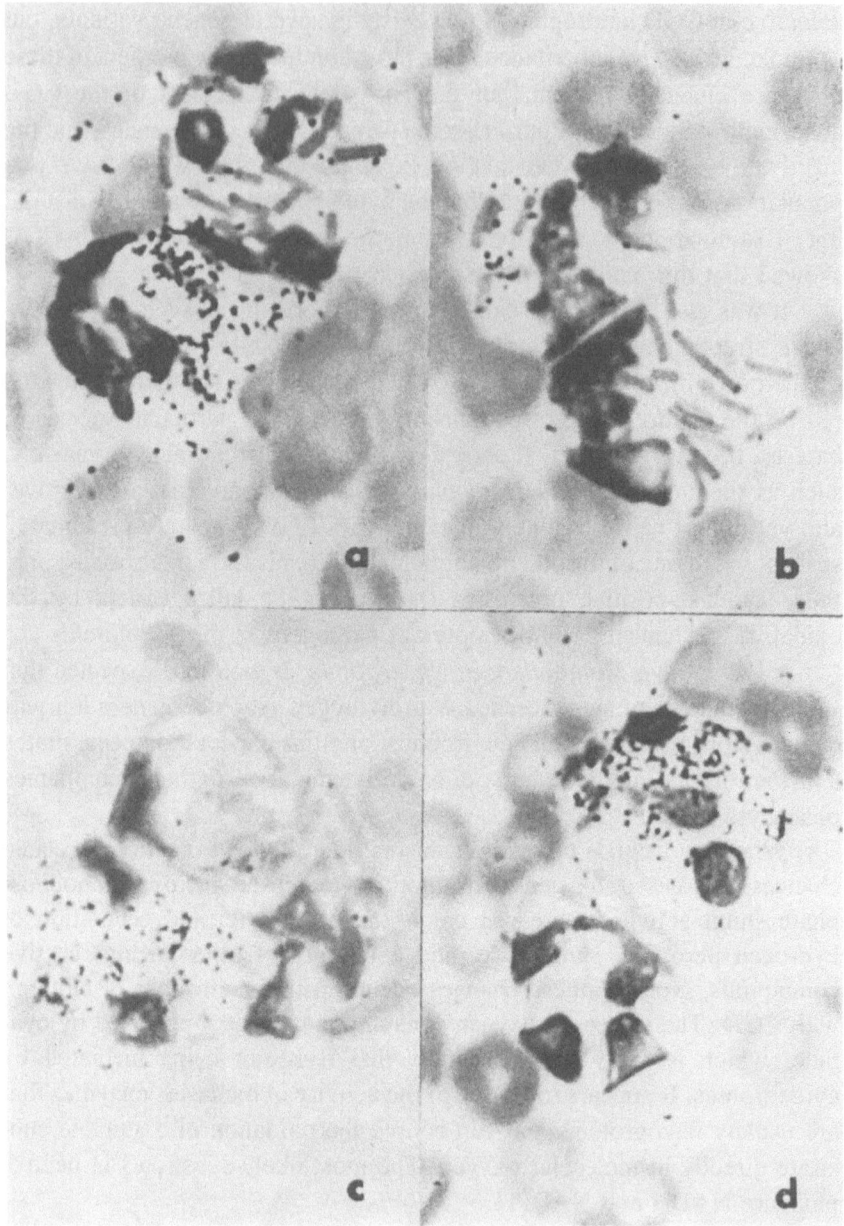

FIG. 7.6. Two populations of neutrophils in the mothers of boys with CGD. One population can iodinate *S. marcescens*, the other cannot. These are four different fields. (From Klebanoff and White.[19])

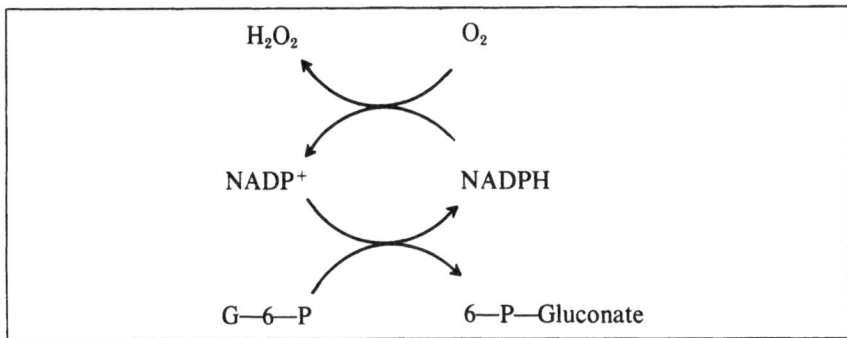

FIG. 7.7. Rossi's scheme for generating hydrogen peroxide by direct oxidation of NADPH.

$NADP^+$, so a two-cycle system could be envisaged (Fig. 7.7). The question of whether the shunt drives the oxidation of NADPH or *vice versa* can be answered very simply: There is no evidence that the quantity or activity of the pentose pathway enzymes is affected by phagocytosis, and therefore the availability of $NADP^+$ must control the activity of the pentose pathway. Formate oxidation is mediated by catalase in the cell sap, and is one of the ways in which the neutrophil can dispose of excess hydrogen peroxide before it rises to dangerous levels. Other pathways are direct decomposition of hydrogen peroxide by catalase, diffusion of hydrogen peroxide out of the cell into the surrounding medium, and consumption of hydrogen peroxide in reactions mediated by myeloperoxidase.

Rossi and his co-workers have evidence for the existence of a KCN-insensitive NADPH oxidase in guinea pig neutrophil granules.[20] The type of granule is unspecified. There is also NADH oxidase activity, but it is smaller in extent. During phagocytosis, both oxidases increase greatly in activity, but the increase in NADPH oxidase is more marked. Activation of the NADPH oxidase can be demonstrated within 30 sec of phagocytosis, and there is a corresponding drop in the concentration of NADPH in the cells. Also, the K_m of NADPH oxidase decreases by about eightfold after phagocytosis. Measurement of the NAD^+:NADH and $NADP^+$:NADPH ratios in living neutrophils at rest and during phagocytosis showed that the former was unchanged, and the latter increased by a factor of three. Rossi believes that the signal for activation of granular NADPH oxidase comes from the plasma membrane, and he showed that detergents, antibodies, and certain other agents acting on the cell surface could trigger oxygen consumption in the absence of phagocytosis. Another such stimulus is phorbol myristic acetate; since this substance is known to induce lysis of the specific granules and the formation of intracytoplasmic vesicles, it would be of great interest to know whether Rossi's enzyme is in the specific granules.

Several American workers doubt that this relatively simple system accounts for the increased oxygen consumption of phagocytosis. There are various technical problems that only experts can solve: What is the most appropriate medium for estimating the activity of these enzymes? (The answers obtained are powerfully influenced by the pH, ionic strength, metal ion content, and other properties of the medium, and no one is really sure what the intracellular environment of the enzymes is.) Would a granular enzyme have access to the highly charged NADPH in the cytoplasm? Are the quantities of enzyme demonstrated really adequate to mediate the observed oxygen consumption? The alternative to an NADPH oxidase is a much more complicated system in which hydrogen peroxide is generated by the oxidation of NADH. NAD^+ cannot be used as cofactor for the first two steps of the hexose monophosphate shunt, so it is necessary to have some mechanism for reducing NAD^+ at the expense of NADPH. It is thought that hydrogen peroxide is used to oxidize glutathione, and that glutathione in turn is reduced by $NADPH^+$ (Fig. 7.8). A less likely possibility is thought to be a transhydrogenase that directly reduces NAD^+ at the expense of NADPH.

The NADH oxidase theory can be criticized because glutathione peroxidase and the $NAD^+/NADPH$ transhydrogenase cannot be demonstrated in the neutrophils of some species. A crucial test that should enable one to distinguish between the alternatives is the respiratory quotient (the ratio between carbon dioxide generated from glucose carbon atom 1 and the oxygen consumed by the cell). The reason is that in scheme 1, there is tight coupling between oxygen consumption and glucose-6-phosphate oxidation. The concentrations of $NADP^+$ and NADPH are so low that they can act only catalytically; no change in the ratio of $NADP^+$ to NADPH could move the respiratory quotient significantly from 1. On the other hand, in scheme 2, there is room for maneuver. Driving the hexose monophosphate shunt is only one of the uses to which hydrogen peroxide can be put. Any peroxide diverted to formate oxidation or reactions involving myeloperoxidase will not stimulate glucose C1 oxidation. The respiratory quotient will thus be low. Furthermore, the immediate result of the glutathione cycle is the oxidation of one molecule of NADPH at the expense of one molecule of hydrogen peroxide. Since two molecules of NADPH are consumed in the oxidation of glucose C1, the respiratory quotient early after phagocytosis will be 0.5. The evidence on this point is in direct

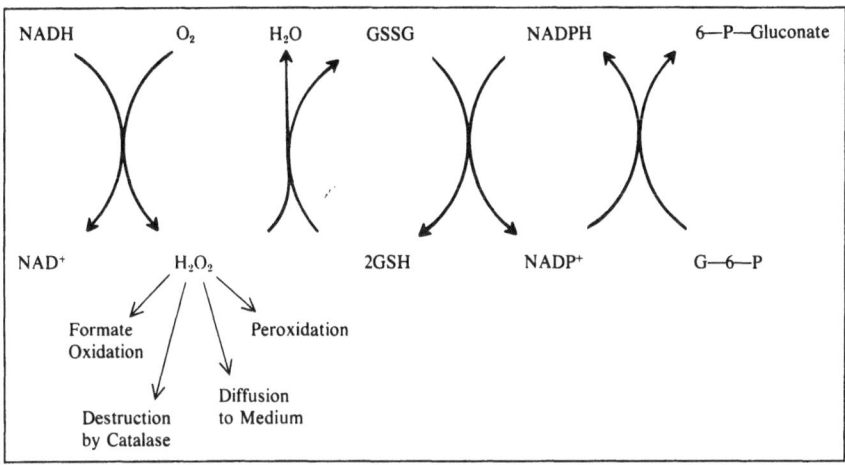

FIG. 7.8. Alternative scheme for generating hydrogen peroxide by oxidation of NADH. Note that hydrogen peroxide can be used in many other ways than driving the hexose monophosphate shunt.

conflict—one set of investigators says that the respiratory quotient is 1, the other that it is much less than 1.[20,21]

Part of the confusion about the importance of NADH oxidase *versus* NADPH oxidase lies in the fact that neither enzyme has been purified. In fact, both oxidations might be mediated by the same molecule, though with different efficiencies. If there are indeed two different enzymes, none of the presently available evidence allows one to make a definitive decision between them. The reason so much interest has been taken in what may seem a trivial point is that an understanding of the enzymatic pathways that generate peroxide will throw light on the pathogenesis of chronic granulomatous disease.

CGD neutrophils have been examined for the presence of all these enzymes. Defects in NADH oxidase, NADPH oxidase, and glutathione peroxidase have all been claimed to be important in particular patients. It is in fact probable that CGD has many causes, and that the defect in the common sex-linked variety is not the same as that in the autosomal recessive, which also affects girls. However, two recent papers make it appear that Rossi is going to carry the day. Both Hohn and Lehrer[22] and Curnutte *et al.*[23] agree that there is a pyridine nucleotide oxidase in the granules of human neutrophils, the activity of which increases six- or eightfold after phagocytosis. In both sets of experiments, NADPH was a much better substrate for the enzyme than was NADH. Granule preparations from CGD neutrophils that had phagocytosed particles showed either no or minimal oxidase activity. There are differences in detail between the experiments, and of course it is still not known whether the defect is absence of the enzyme or inability to activate it. But it does look as though the normal route to hydrogen peroxide formation is via the oxidation of NADPH.

(c) Superoxide, Singlet Oxygen, and Free Radicals. Oxidase enzymes do not necessarily or even usually mediate two-electron transfers and form H_2O_2 directly. Their reactions often proceed by one-electron transfer steps that result in the formation of unstable and highly reactive intermediates. In neutrophils, there is evidence of varying quality for the generation of superoxide, singlet oxygen, and the hydroxyl radical.

Superoxide is oxygen that has accepted one electron (Fig. 7.9) It is usually measured by its reduction of cytochrome C, and it will also directly reduce the yellow dye nitroblue tetrazolium (NBT) to a blue insoluble product. Two superoxide molecules can interact with each other to generate hydrogen peroxide and oxygen:

$$2O_2^- + 2H^+ \rightarrow H_2O_2 + O_2$$

Fridovich and his co-workers discovered that virtually all tissues contain an enzyme, superoxide dismutase, that catalyzes this reaction.[24] Bacteria also have superoxide dismutases, and it is of some interest that gram-negative organisms have two enzymes, one in the cytoplasm and one in the periplasmic space. The first is apparently to protect them against superoxide they produce themselves, and the second to protect them against superoxide coming in from the medium. Strictly anaerobic bacteria do not possess dismutases; it has been suggested that this lack is the reason they are anaerobic.

Normal neutrophils engaged in phagocytosis reduce NBT and secrete into the medium something that reduces cytochrome C. Both these reac-

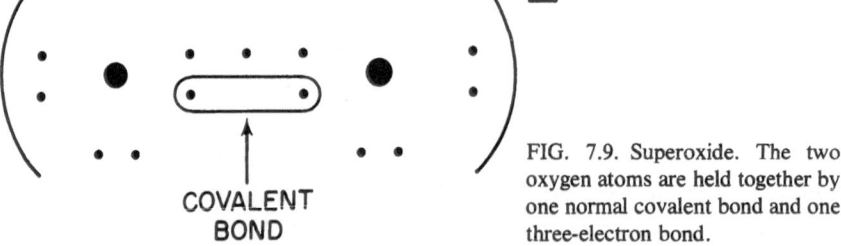

COVALENT
BOND

FIG. 7.9. Superoxide. The two oxygen atoms are held together by one normal covalent bond and one three-electron bond.

(a)

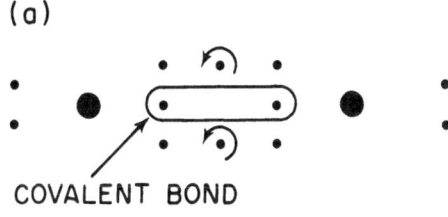

COVALENT BOND

FIG. 7.10.(a) The oxygen molecule in its normal (triplet) state. There is one covalent bond and two three-electron bonds. The unpaired electron spins are parallel. (b) Singlet oxygen. The unpaired electron spins are in opposition. The energy released by decay to the normal state is 37.8 kcal/mol. (Figs. 7.9 and 7.10 based on Pauling, L., *The Nature of the Chemical Bond*, 3rd ed., Cornell University Press, 1960.)

(b)

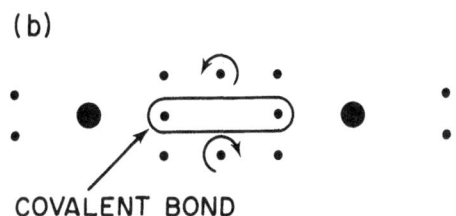

COVALENT BOND

tions are antagonized by superoxide dismutase, and are therefore presumably mediated by superoxide.[25]

Singlet oxygen is an electronically excited state of oxygen that spontaneously decays to the normal triplet state with emission of a photon of red light (Fig. 7.10). It is thought to be generated in neutrophils, because flashes of light do in fact occur when neutrophils are fed organisms. The flashes are too weak to see, but they can be counted in a scintillation counter with the coincidence circuit turned off.[26] The most plausible mechanism for light production is a reaction involving myeloperoxidase, hydrogen peroxide, and chloride—a reaction that also exhibits chemiluminescence, that involves components available in neutrophils, and that is thought to be important in bacterial killing. However, Webb found that the chemiluminescence of neutrophils was inhibited by superoxide dismutase,[27] so there are other possibilities. Light production by neutrophils is maximal about 15 min after ingestion of organisms, which is about the time when azurophil granules have maximally degranulated. Singlet oxygen can combine across the double bonds of unsaturated fatty acids, and it has been suggested that this might kill microorganisms.

The hydroxyl radical, ·OH, is a very strong oxidizing agent, and can interact with unsaturated fatty acids to yield malondialdehyde. Such peroxidative changes have been demonstrated in the membranes of phagocytic vesicles.[28] Hydroxyl radical may be generated as follows:

$$O_2^- + H_2O_2 \rightarrow \cdot OH + OH^- + O_2$$

7.4.3. Oxidative Killing of Bacteria

How are all these oxidative products that are developed in neutrophils used to kill bacteria? At the present moment, much noise is being made about the importance of superoxide and the other reactive substances. However, the only product that has been unequivocally shown to kill microorganisms at present is hydrogen peroxide, and the most efficient way of using it to kill bacteria is in combination with the myeloperoxidase of azurophil granules. Exactly how bacteria are killed is not certain. The system is most effective at a pH of about 5, which is attained in phagocytic vacuoles. When iodine is the oxidizable halide, it is fixed into bacterial proteins, and this was originally thought to be the mechanism. It may be, however, that some other oxidation is the lethal event, and iodination is peripheral.

When chloride is the halide, it is not substituted into bacterial proteins, and yet bacteria are efficiently killed. The $MPO-H_2O_2-Cl^-$ system can oxidatively deaminate and decarboxylate amino acids. It is thought that hypochlorous acid is formed by the $MPO-H_2O_2$ complex, and that this acid reacts with amino acids to generate chloramines. These chloramines decompose spontaneously, with the liberation of carbon dioxide, ammonia, and Cl^-, and the truncated amino acid skeleton is left with an aldehyde group. Formaldehyde and glutaraldehyde are well-known disinfectants, and other aldehydes share this property. However, it is not likely that generation of aldehydes from free amino acids in vesicle contents is the bactericidal mechanism, because *in vitro,* the addition of alanine actually inhibits the killing of bacteria by $MPO-H_2O_2-Cl^-$. Rather, it would seem that some substrate on the bacterium itself must be oxidized. This view was confirmed by some experiments by Paul and his colleagues, who showed that if *E. coli* was separated from $MPO-H_2O_2-Cl^-$ by a dialysis membrane, no killing occurred. Hypochlorous acid itself could cross the dialysis membrane and kill the bacteria.[29]

Iodide cannot mediate decarboxylation and deamination of amino acids, so the bactericidal reaction must be something else. This view is supported by the effects of taurine, which forms a stable chloramine when acted on by $MPO-H_2O_2-Cl^-$. This compound blocks killing of bacteria by $MPO-H_2O_2-Cl^-$, but not by $MPO-H_2O_2-I^-$.[29]

The primary importance of $MPO-H_2O_2$ systems in killing bacteria is supported by much indirect evidence, such as the defect in CGD neutrophils and failure to kill under anaerobic conditions. However, these defects could also be viewed as due to failure to generate superoxide or some other reactive compound. Azide, cyanide, and propylthiouracil are inhibitors of peroxidase, but do not interfere with hydrogen peroxide formation. All are effective inhibitors of bacterial killing within neutrophils. Killing is not totally abolished, however, whereas iodination is. This is one reason for believing that iodination *per se* may not be the cause of bacterial death. Klebanoff showed that a system composed of xanthine, xanthine oxidase, myeloperoxidase, and chloride was strongly bactericidal for *E. coli*. Xanthine plus xanthine oxidase generates superoxide, which gives rise to various products, including the hydroxyl radical and hydrogen peroxide. The bactericidal activity of the system was almost abolished by catalase. Since catalase has no action on O_2^- or $\cdot OH$, it seemed likely that these radicals were not playing a major role in bacterial killing.[30] Another piece of evidence that strongly suggests hydrogen peroxide, and not some free radical, is responsible for killing bacteria is Root's observation that the bactericidal defect of CGD neutrophils can be reversed by supplying exogenous hydrogen peroxide.[21] Killing of staphylococci at 1 hr was perhaps a little defective, but at 2 hr, it was unequivocally normal.

7.4.4. Oxidative Killing Mechanisms Not Involving Peroxidase

In view of all this evidence, it was a very unpleasant surprise when Lehrer and Cline reported a patient nearly 50 years of age whose neutrophils were totally defective in myeloperoxidase.[31] The patient was in trouble with a *Candida albicans* infection, and it was shown that his neutrophils were indeed incapable of killing this organism. But the patient's age was a guarantee of reasonable antibacterial defenses, and sure enough, staphylococci were killed in his neutrophils, though at a subnormal rate. About a dozen such patients are now known; most of the rest are in perfect health. Also, Spitznagel has shown that the neutrophils of the chicken and certain other species have no peroxidase whatever.

The explanation appears to be that hydrogen peroxide can participate in bactericidal reactions that are not mediated by myeloperoxidase. MPO-deficient cells develop much more hydrogen peroxide than normal cells, because they lack a major pathway for disposing of it. Their ability to kill staphylococci is seriously impaired under anaerobic conditions, suggesting that hydrogen peroxide is needed for the reaction. The most attractive candidate for this mechanism at present is that described by Miller, which involves the simultaneous action of ascorbic acid (vitamin C), hydrogen peroxide, and lysozyme.[32] Ascorbate is a powerful reducing agent, and hydrogen peroxide a powerful oxidizing agent; Miller thought it likely that free radicals were generated, damaged the bacterial cell wall, and allowed lysozyme access to its substrate in the basal layer. Karnovsky investigated this system further, and found that ascorbate and hydrogen peroxide were bactericidal by themselves if either cobalt or copper was added.[33] Copper plus hydrogen peroxide plus dehydroascorbate was even more effective. Free-radical scavengers such as thiosulfate inhibit some of these systems, but which radical or radicals are involved is not known. Ascorbate, hydrogen peroxide, copper, cobalt, and lysozyme are all present in neutrophils; whether they can all be brought together in the phagocytic vesicle is not known.

Another possible bactericidal mechanism utilizing hydrogen peroxide involves D-amino acid oxidase. D-Amino acids are part of the peptidoglycan layer of the cell wall of all bacteria, but they are not found in mammalian tissues. Lehrer and Cline showed that neutrophil granules (type not specified) contained D-amino acid oxidase, and that this oxidase could oxidize D-amino acid residues in bacterial cell walls with generation of hydrogen peroxide. By itself, this reaction was only moderately bactericidal, but it did kill over two-thirds of an inoculum of *E. coli* in 30 min.[34]

It seems likely that most if not all the cellular hydrogen peroxide is generated by the dismutation of superoxide. Therefore, if hydrogen peroxide is the major bactericidal substance, one would expect that the addition of superoxide dismutase (SD) to a suspension of neutrophils and bacteria would if anything enhance microbial killing. But Johnston *et al.* have evidence that bactericidal activity is in fact somewhat diminished by the addition of SD, especially if it is covalently coupled to the surface of a particle, and thus is carried straight into the phagocytic vacuole.[35] This is suggestive evidence that superoxide is perhaps involved in bacterial killing in its own right. However, the evidence is far from conclusive, and there is really no hard evidence that other active substances such as singlet oxygen or the hydroxyl radical are necessary for bacterial killing.

7.4.5. Nonoxidative Bactericidal Mechanisms

The neutrophil bactericidal mechanisms that are not dependent on oxygen are somewhat in the background at present because of the spectacular progress being made in the understanding of the oxidative ones. And yet, only two families of bacteria require oxygen for killing; the rest are disposed of perfectly well in nitrogen.[15] Most of these bacteria are "non-pathogenic," but one would suppose that the reason is merely that the neutrophil has efficient methods for disposing of them. Spitznagel discovered that chicken neutrophils are totally deficient in myeloperoxidase,[36] and furthermore that they do not appear even to produce hydrogen peroxide after phagocytosis.[37] Needless to say, chickens have no unusual susceptibility to infection, and in fact, their neutrophils can kill a variety of organisms perfectly well. It is not yet known whether they require oxygen to do so. It is known that their granules contain two different types of lysozyme, and bactericidal cationic proteins analogous to those discussed below.

Unfortunately, there is no well-known clinical deficiency state that underlines the importance of nonoxidative bactericidal mechanisms, and much less is known about the details of their action. However, from the teleological point of view, specific granules would hardly have evolved and come to predominate in mature neutrophils unless they served a function. And the only well-established function of neutrophils is to kill bacteria.

(a) pH and Lactic Acid. Lactic acid is generated in large quantities during phagocytosis because of the increased glycolytic activity. In some unknown way, the excess hydrogen ions are concentrated in phagocytic vesicles. Bainton covalently coupled yeast particles to various pH indicator dyes, allowed them to be phagocytosed, and watched the color changes.[38] Within 3 min of uptake, the pH dropped to 6.5 or below, as assessed by neutral red; by 7–15 min, the pH had reached 4.0, as assessed by bromcresol green. It did not fall much below 4.0, because bromophenol blue did not change color at any time. Few bacteria can continue to grow at pH 4.0, and many are actually killed by lactic acid in low concentration. However, it is not known whether lactate also enters phagocytic vesicles, and perhaps the main effect of the change in pH is to facilitate the action of myeloperoxidase and other granular enzymes.

(b) Lysozyme. Lysozyme kills those few gram-positive bacteria that do not have some covering for their peptidoglycan layer. However, it can kill many gram-positive and gram-negative organisms if some other agent damages the cell wall and allows lysozyme access to its substrate. One of the damaging agents that seems likely to be important is antibody and complement.[39] There is clear evidence of synergy among antibody, complement, and lysozyme for the most diverse organisms; even the tubercle bacillus may be killed by the combination. Furthermore, there is evidence for many organisms that bacteria opsonized by amounts of antibody and

complement that are adequate to ensure phagocytosis are not always killed within the cells. Increasing the amount of complement does lead to intracellular death,[40] and while one does not know that lysozyme was responsible, it would be consistent with the *in vitro* data. Chelating agents can also synergize with lysozyme, and it may be worth remembering that lactoferrin can bind metal ions other than Fe^{3+}. Finally, Brumfitt and Glynn found an organism the intracellular death or survival of which appeared to be entirely determined by whether or not it was susceptible to lysozyme.[41] They took a strain of *Micrococcus lysodeikticus* and grew it on plates containing lysozyme. Lysozyme-resistant variants grew out, and by progressive increase in the concentration of lysozyme in the plates, they obtained a variant that was more than 40,000 times more resistant to lysozyme that the parent strain. This organism was phagocytosed normally by human neutrophils, but was not killed appreciably in a period of 1 hr, whereas much less than 1% of the parent strain remained alive. The mechanism of the resistance was known to be acetylation of the cell wall; removal of the acetyl groups by treatment with glycine at pH 11 had no effect on the viability of the organisms, but rendered them completely susceptible to destruction within neutrophils.

This organism must have been resistant to the oxidative bactericidal mechanisms of neutrophils, and proves that this resistance is possible. However, it was not particularly pathogenic for mice, even when injected intracerebrally. One reason might have been that the lysozyme-resistant variant was exceedingly slow to grow.

(c) Lactoferrin. As far as is known, lactoferrin by itself is merely bacteriostatic. Nonetheless, it may constitute 10% of the total protein of the cell, and one has the feeling that this must be purposive. It seems probable that lactoferrin synergizes with something else, but virtually no experiments along this line have been performed. One observation that may be relevant is that killing of gram-negative organisms by antibody and complement in normal serum can be completely inhibited by adding a ferric salt. This salt saturates the serum transferrin, which normally holds the free Fe^{3+} concentration of serum at very low levels.[42] The initial effect of antibody and complement on a gram-negative organism is to stop RNA synthesis abruptly. Cessation of DNA and protein synthesis, and gross alterations in cell membrane permeability, occur only after a considerable delay. If the medium contains enough iron to saturate the transferrin, the initial check of RNA synthesis still occurs, but bacterial growth resumes after a couple of hours. Something chelated by transferrin is clearly impor-

TABLE 7.1. Activities of Cationic Proteins (Purified by Sucrose Density
Gradient Electrophoresis) Against Several Genera of Bacteria

[The initial concentration was 1×10^6 organisms/ml, and the organisms were incubated with the cationic proteins for 1 hr at pH 5.6 and 37°C. The quantity of each fraction that reduced bacterial growth by 50% was taken as 1 unit; activities were expressed as units/mg protein. Note that this assay does not measure bacterial death. Modified from Zeya, H. I., and Spitznagel, J. K., *J. Exp. Med.* 127:927 (1968).]

Test bacteria	Cationic protein fraction					
	I	II	III	IV	V	VI (Lysozyme)
Staphylococcus aureus	—	—	600	—	—	120
Staphylococcus albus	—	—	600	—	—	—
Streptococcus faecalis	500	500	300	4000	800	250
Proteus vulgaris	—	—	—	—	900	200
Escherichia coli 0117:H27	400	400	—	—	200	—

tant to nucleic acid metabolism in gram-negative bacteria, and the same may be true of lactoferrin.

(d) Cationic Proteins. The chemical nature and specificity of phagocytin were worked out by Zeya and Spitznagel.[43] They were able to overcome its instability by lysing granules at the origin of an electrophoretic strip and immediately separating the constituent proteins by turning on the current. "Phagocytin" moved toward the cathode at pH 8.6, and proved to be a family of basic proteins with isoelectric points above 11 and containing a great deal of arginine. By sucrose density gradient electrophoresis, they were able to achieve higher resolution, and found that the cationic proteins showed some specificity of bactericidal effect. Thus, the fastest-migrating components (I and II) killed *Streptococcus faecalis; Staphylococcus aureus* was killed by Component III, and *Proteus vulgaris* by Component V. In each case, the other fractions were ineffective. Other bacteria were susceptible to more than one fraction, though the amounts of protein required to kill might vary markedly. Sometimes, different strains of the same organism varied in their susceptibility; thus, *E. coli* B was easily killed by Component IV, while *E. coli* 0117:H27, 026–B6, and K12 were entirely unaffected (Table 7.1).

Olsson has recently extended these studies, using human neutrophils.[44] Several cationic antibacterial proteins were found; however, they had very similar amino acid compositions and were all neutralized by an antibody raised against one of them. The cationic proteins were confined to azurophil granules.[45] Their pH optimum was near neutrality; this finding is of interest, because most of the proteolytic enzymes of human neutrophil granules also have a pH optimum near neutrality. Furthermore, Mandell found that human neutrophils, as distinct from rat, mouse, and rabbit neutrophils, developed an intravacuolar pH of only 6.0–6.5 following phagocytosis.[46] If this is so, then cationic proteins would have good opportunity to be active in human neutrophils, and may well be an important cause of bacterial death.

Nothing is known about the mechanism of bacterial killing by these proteins. It is worth noting that many other strongly basic proteins can also kill bacteria without lysing them. One would expect such proteins to stick to bacterial surfaces, which in general are negatively charged. However, it is not clear why this sticking should be lethal. There is a precedent for bacterial killing by adsorption of a specific protein to the cell wall, without entry of the protein into the cell. Certain *E. coli* strains make proteins, the colicines, that can kill other *E. coli* strains in this way.

(e) Defects in Specific Granules. There are now reports of scattered patients with unusual infections that have been attributed to the absence of specific granules. However, no two of the patients have been entirely comparable, and only one appears to have had a truly congenital defect. In his case, the specific granules were very few, very small, and morphologically abnormal.[47] However, there were also abnormalities of nuclear segmentation, and the cells did not possess alkaline phosphatase. Since alkaline phosphatase is now known not to occur in specific granules, it is clear that several defects are involved in this boy, and it is not clear that the abnormality in the specific granules is the cause of his recurrent staphylococcal infections.

Spitznagel did describe a man whose neutrophils were completely deficient in specific granules and were unable to kill several species of bacteria.[48] The man was said to be susceptible to infection; however, he was 43, so the defect was certainly not diastrous, and to date he remains an isolated case.

Neutrophils thus contain an array of bactericidal mechanisms, and it seems probable that important ones remain to be discovered. For most organisms, there is a great "overkill" capacity, in that any one of several bactericidal mechanisms would serve to kill them. Chronic granulomatous disease is the most obvious example of a defect that cannot be adequately compensated for. Yet even in this case, there is substantial evidence of intracellular killing of the organisms that cause clinical problems in these patients. Root found, for example, that normal neutrophils killed more than

95% of staphylococci over 2 hr. In the same time, CGD neutrophils killed about 70%.[21] Plainly, this percentage of killing is inadequate in the long run, but it does mean that the other mechanisms are not totally ineffective. Presumably, this is why even CGD is not so devastating as total absence of neutrophils.

7.5. Summary

When bacteria are phagocytosed by neutrophils, each is enclosed in a vacuole bounded by an area of membrane that was originally located on the surface of the cell. There is no communication between the vacuole and the neutrophil cytoplasm. The granules are also membrane-bound, and after phagocytosis, their membranes fuse with the membranes of the phagocytic vacuole, so that granular proteins are discharged directly onto the surface of the bacterium.

Some of these granular proteins are directly bactericidal or bacteriostatic. They include lysozyme, which hydrolyzes a mucopeptide found in the cell wall of all bacteria; lactoferrin, which denies bacteria the iron they need to grow; and cationic proteins, which are a family of highly basic proteins that inhibit or kill bacteria in unknown ways.

A very important mechanism for killing bacteria depends on the generation of hydrogen peroxide by the neutrophil. This generation requires the availability of molecular oxygen, which is used to oxidize a pyridine nucleotide, with the production of hydrogen peroxide. Details of this process are still obscure, but it seems that the most important nucleotide is NADPH, and that the oxidase is located in the granules, becoming activated after phagocytosis. In the presence of either I^- or Cl^-, myeloperoxidase from azurophil granules can use hydrogen peroxide to kill bacteria. The generation of hydrogen peroxide is defective in chronic granulomatous disease, which accounts both for the increased susceptibility to infection and for the fact that only certain organisms are troublesome in these patients.

Other chemically reactive substances, such as superoxide, singlet oxygen, and the hydroxyl radical, are generated during NADPH oxidation. At present, it is not known whether any of these are important except as generators of hydrogen peroxide.

There is evidence that hydrogen peroxide can mediate bacterial killing in neutrophils that are totally deficient in myeloperoxidase; the mechanisms are uncertain, but appear to involve cooperation among several factors. It seems likely that in the restricted volume of a phagocytic vacuole, synergy among mechanisms that are individually weak is common. In particular, the amount of complement fixed on the surface of a bacterium may affect its intracellular fate.

8

Other Activities of Neutrophils

It is perfectly clear that the principal function of neutrophils is to kill bacteria. However, the enzymes they contain are capable of killing and breaking down all living tissue, and under some circumstances, neutrophils are responsible for considerable damage to the host. In bacterial infections, this damage is usually expressed by abscess formation. There is also a series of responses and conditions that are not primarily infective in origin, but in which for one reason or another neutrophil enzymes are let loose in tissue and damage or destroy it. The series includes serum sickness, the Arthus reaction, and the Shwartzmann reaction, and such clinical conditions as gout, probably rheumatoid arthritis, and several types of glomerulonephritis.

In the past, various activities in aseptically injured tissue have been ascribed to neutrophils. Thus, they have been thought to aid in the breakdown of dead tissue in infarcts, in the disposal of erythrocytes in hematomas, and in the healing of wounds. These opinions were based largely on the fact that neutrophils were present in such lesions, that they were phagocytic, and a vague feeling that these activities ought to be useful. At present, only scanty direct evidence is available, but it would suggest that the role of neutrophils in tissue repair has been exaggerated.

Finally, there is a group of responses to infection or inflammation that appear to be due to substances secreted by neutrophils in the local lesions. These substances get into the bloodstream, either directly or through lymphatics, and influence the function of distant tissues. The best-known example of such a response is fever; others include the increased synthesis of fibrinogen, haptoglobins, and ceruloplasmin by the liver; the sequestration of iron and zinc in the reticuloendothelial system; and the mobilization of neutrophils by bone marrow. It is possible that all these activities are mediated by the same substance.

8.1. Extracellular Release of Neutrophil Granule Contents

8.1.1. Enzyme Release During Phagocytosis

In describing the degranulation phenomenon, Cohn and Hirsh observed that small quantities of hydrolytic enzymes, less than 10% of the total available in the cell, were released to the external medium during phagocytosis.[1] They were measuring enzymes that we now know to be contained in azurophil granules, and we also know that azurophil granules are rather slow to fuse with phagocytic vacuoles. Weissman showed that the probable mechanism for extracellular release of enzymes is fusion of granules with phagocytic vacuoles that have not yet closed.[2] If this is the mechanism, one would predict that extracellular release of the contents of specific granules would occur to a much greater extent, because they fuse earlier than do azurophil granules. One would also predict that phagocytosis of large particles would be more likely to lead to extracellular release of enzymes than phagocytosis of small ones.

These predictions have been verified by several workers. It has been shown that phagocytosis of yeast particles (2–4 μm) leads to more extracellular release than phagocytosis of staphylococci (1 μm). Remember that a particle with a diameter of 3 μm is 27 times bigger than one with a diameter of 1 μm. A more quantitative study by Henson involved the use of latex particles of 2, 1, 0.5, and 0.1 μm diameter. The particles were opsonized with IgG, and equal quantities of IgG were presented to neutrophils. The amounts of β-glucuronidase released to the medium were 22, 19, 16, and 9%, respectively.[3] Antigen–antibody complexes are a particularly effective stimulus for extracellular release; whether this is because of their size or for some other reason is unclear. Using human neutrophils and antigen–antibody complexes, Leffell and Spitznagel found that over 90% of the lactoferrin in the cells was released to the medium, and nearly 50% of the myeloperoxidase. These are markers for specific and azurophil granules, respectively.[4]

8.1.2. Enzyme Release During "Frustrated Phagocytosis"

The logical result of increasing particle size without limit would be that the neutrophil would be unable to phagocytose the object, and would spread out along it and degranulate directly onto its surface. This occurrence was demonstrated by Henson, who captured antigen–antibody complexes on the surface of a micropore filter and then drew a suspension of neutrophils gently down onto the filter surface.[5] External degranulation was demonstrated by electron microscopy, as well as by quantitating the amounts of granular enzymes released. One interesting finding of this study was that very small quantities of antigen–antibody complexes on filters would lead to large amounts of extracellular enzyme release. In one case, 2 μg of complexes on a filter was as effective as 30 μg in free suspension. Another finding of interest concerned alkaline phosphatase, which at the time was thought to be a marker for specific granules. Henson found, as had others, that little of the enzyme was released extracellularly, but he showed that it was incorporated into the walls of phagocytic vesicles and into the external cell membrane when the complex could not be phagocytosed. Thus, at least three distinguishable cell organelles undergo a membrane-fusion process with phagocytic vacuoles.

Last, Henson investigated the ability of neutrophils to adhere to and to degranulate in response to immunoglobulins of different classes in the absence of complement.[6] There is a type of tumor known as *myeloma,* in which a single clone of plasma cells multiplies until it has replaced much of the bone marrow and also grows extensively as nodules in the liver, spleen, and other organs. These malignant cells produce a single immunoglobulin molecule that eventually constitutes the major part of the serum protein and can be isolated in a reasonably homogeneous state. Each tumor produces a different immunoglobulin, and by processing serum from many separate patients, a range of pure immunoglobulin molecules of different classes can be obtained. Such immunoglobulins are known as *myeloma proteins,* and were used by Henson in this study.

He found that neutrophils would phagocytose aggregated IgG of any of the four subclasses, and also aggregated IgA. Aggregated IgD or IgM was ineffective. Aggregated immunoglobulins on membranes were much more efficient, but even on membranes, aggregated IgD or IgM led to no more extracellular enzyme release than did bovine serum albumin. Complement was not present in these experiments, so it would appear that neutrophils must have more "receptors" than were apparent from the rosetting techniques discussed in Chapter 5.

Since a number of the conditions to be discussed involved the deposition of antigen–antibody complexes on membranes within the body, it seems likely that Henson's work is of biological as well as theoretical importance.

8.1.3. Enzyme Release Stimulated by Chemotactic Factors

Goldstein and his co-workers have shown that neutrophils can be stimulated to release enzymes extracellularly in the absence of particulate matter.[7] They activated the alternate complement pathway of human serum by treatment with yeast particles or a factor from cobra venom. Serum so activated contained something, probably C5a, that stimulated enzyme release from neutrophils paralyzed with cytochalasin B. Since this situation is highly artificial, it may not be relevant *in vivo*, but Becker has independent evidence that lysosomal enzyme release may be triggered by chemotactic factors. He used C3a, C5a, C5b,6,7, and a bacterial chemotactic factor from *E. coli*. None of these substances caused enzyme release from neutrophils in free suspension, but all would do so if the neutrophils were on a membrane with pore size greater than 0.6 μm. Why it was necessary for the cells to be able to enter the membrane was not clear, but it was suggested that the process was another example of the response of neutrophils to a nonphagocytoseable surface.[8] One wonders whether this triggering of lysosomal enzyme release by neutrophils responding to chemotactic factors and engaged in negotiating a narrow passageway has anything to do with their ability to emigrate from blood vessels in inflamed tissue.

8.1.4. Enzyme Release After Cell Death

Another mechanism for release of neutrophil enzymes is the death of the cell. This death presumably occurs in all tissues to some degree, as neutrophils reach the end of their allotted span and disintegrate. In inflamed tissue, there are many more neutrophils, and this release from senescent cells will be exaggerated. In addition, there are factors in inflamed areas that would be expected to positively kill cells. Many bacteria secrete into the medium enzymes that damage cell membranes. Examples are the streptolysins O and S, the leukocidin of *Staphylococcus aureus,* the phospholipase C of *Pseudomonas aeruginosa,* and the α toxin of *Clostridium perfringens*. The amounts of these toxins produced by individual organisms appear to be inconsequential, because dilute suspensions of almost any adequately opsonized bacterium are taken up and destroyed by neutrophils. However, once large local populations have built up, these substances may become very important; certainly, it can be seen that neutrophils migrating toward an abscess cavity die before they reach it. Sterile dead tissue also seems to produce something that kills neutrophils; most of the neutrophils around infarcts have pyknotic nuclei.

8.1.5. Cell Lysis from Within

Finally, neutrophil enzymes may be released to the exterior because the cell has been undone from within. The purest example of this phenomenon is in gout, in which urate crystals form in joint fluid and are phagocytosed by neutrophils. Shirahama and Cohen mixed urate crystals with various electron-microscopic markers, allowed neutrophils to phagocytose the mixtures, and took samples for electron microscopy at intervals.[9] The markers were thorotrast, colloidal carbon, ferritin, and horseradish peroxidase; similar results were obtained with all of them. At 5 min, urate crystals plus the tracers had been taken up and were enclosed in phagocytic vacuoles. However, at 30 min, the membranes of the phagocytic vacuoles showed defects, and the tracers had leaked out into the cytoplasm. By 60 min, most of the neutrophils were unequivocally dead, with grossly disorganized vacuolated cytoplasm, rupture of the cytoplasmic membrane, and liberation of tracers into the external medium again.

This lysis from within is also seen in silicosis and after phagocytosis of *Streptococcus pyogenes*. In the latter case, the lysis appears to be mediated by streptolysin S; why urate and silica lead to membrane lysis is not known. The result is that the neutrophil is digested by its own enzymes, and when the cell dies, the enzymes are liberated into the external medium.

8.2. Enzymes Responsible for Tissue Damage

8.2.1. Cathepsins

Having considered the circumstances under which neutrophils release their granular contents extracellularly, we could reasonably discuss just which enzymes are responsible for damaging living tissue. This discussion is far from easy, however, because so many enzymes are involved, and there is much uncertainty about the conditions under which they operate *in vivo*. Most lysosomal enzymes have maximal activity at a low pH, as low as 2.5–3 in some cases. At first sight, that would appear to disqualify them for any extracellular role, since the pH in living tissue is 7.35 or thereabouts. However, we do not know what the pH may be at the interface between a spread-out neutrophil and a vascular basement membrane on which lie antigen–antibody complexes. If neutrophils can secrete hydrogen ions into intracellular phagocytic vesicles, there seems to be no reason why the same process could not occur into granule membranes that happen to have fused with the cell membrane. Furthermore, many lysosomal enzymes produce strong acids by acting on their substrates; thus, sulfatases and phosphatases cause liberation of sulfuric and phosphoric acids, respectively. It is therefore possible that the activity of such hydrolytic enzymes could create conditions in which other hydrolases could function. Last, lysosomes may not be membranous bags filled with soluble enzymes that simply await release. Many enzymes may be closely bound to the membrane surface by noncovalent bonds, and this binding may profoundly influence the apparent pH of their environment. In general, enzymes bound to membranes behave as if they were at a pH about 2 units less than that of the surrounding medium. If this rule of thumb applies to cathepsins, they would be maximally active when the external pH was about 6, which does not seem impossible.

It would therefore be unwise to rule out the involvement of the classic lysosomal enzymes in tissue damage. Neutrophil granules contain at least eight proteolytic enzymes with optimal activity at acid pH that collectively are able to break down proteins into individual amino acids. Cathepsins D and E are probably the most important, because they are endopeptidases that can attack native proteins such as hemoglobin and albumin. The fragments can then be further catabolized by other cathepsins that are unable to attack native proteins. Cochrane and Aiken demonstrated that either cathepsin D or cathepsin E could degrade purified glomerular basement membrane if incubated with it at acid pH.[10] There was little or no activity at neutral pH, but as discussed above, the local pH in vessel walls or glomeruli may be quite low.

There is also substantial evidence that cathepsin D may retain some activity in body fluids at a pH that is close to physiological. Neutrophil extracts can liberate from a substrate found in plasma or tissue fluids a kinin that is distinct from bradykinin. There is also a factor that can be extracted from lymph nodes and causes inflammation when injected into the skin.

Both these activities appear to be attributable to cathepsin D. Cathepsin D is also strongly suspected to be the cause of liquefaction and breakdown in tuberculous lesions, and of the breakdown of articular cartilage in certain forms of arthritis.

Cathepsin D has now been purified from several sources, and specific antibody is available. In addition, a fairly specific inhibitor, pepstatin, has been isolated from an actinomycete. With the use of these reagents, it should soon be possible to work out how important cathepsin D really is in causing damage in tissue.

Another enzyme that has maximal activity at pH 5 or less, and that nevertheless demonstrably functions extracellularly, is myeloperoxidase. In 1974, it was shown that when neutrophils phagocytose particles in the presence of ^{125}I, serum proteins in the medium become iodinated.[11] The extent of the iodination was greater when large particles had to be taken up, which suggested that the peroxidase was getting out through open phagocytic vesicles. The presence of peroxidase in the medium was confirmed by showing that the cell-free supernate would iodinate proteins if a source of H_2O_2 was provided. Recently, Klebanoff has shown that neutrophils phagocytosing zymosan can secrete enough extracellular myeloperoxidase to kill unsensitized tumor cells in the same medium.[12] There are also reports of neutrophils killing antibody-coated tumor cells by this mechanism. It is not usual to regard neutrophils as an important defense against tumors, but these experiments do open up some interesting possibilities.

8.2.2. Neutral Proteases

The neutral proteases of neutrophil granules are, as the name suggests, maximally active at physiological pH. The two best known are elastase and collagenase; both have recently been purified, and both appear to be contained in azurophil granules.[13] Elastase has a pH optimum of about 8, but it retains 50% of its activity down to pH 6. It has the unusual ability to hydrolyze long chains of small aliphatic amino acids such as alanine and glycine. These amino acids are common in elastin, which is hardly attacked by any other mammalian proteolytic enzyme. The enzyme is therefore known as *elastase,* but it is in reality a powerful general proteolytic enzyme with activity on many substrates. It exists as three isozymes, which are immunologically indistinguishable, and its action is antagonized by two proteins found in all normal sera: α_1-antitrypsin and α_2-macroglobulin.[14]

Elastase can be selectively inhibited by several synthetic peptides that have been designed to seek out its active site and bind there covalently, thus destroying its activity stoichiometrically. The most efficient is *N*-acetyl–L-ala–L-ala–L-ala-chloromethyl ketone. The (L-ala)₃ chain is a preferred substrate, and the chloromethyl ketone binds covalently to an amino acid residue near the active site, probably histidine. Crude neutrophil granule extracts at neutral pH can digest glomerular basement membrane, articular cartilage, the elastic tissue in arterial walls, and the elastin from lung. If these extracts were treated with the inhibitor, they were still able to digest glomerular basement membrane and articular cartilage, but totally unable to digest the elastin-containing materials. Thus, elastase is one of several granule proteases that are active at neutral pH, but it is the only enzyme that can digest blood-vessel walls.[15]

There is substantial evidence that elastase is important *in vivo*. Injections of purified elastase into the wall of the dog aorta caused breakdown of the elastic tissue at the injection site. Injection into normal rabbit skin led to disruption of small-blood-vessel walls and obvious local hemorrage.[16] In serum sickness, antigen–antibody complexes accumulate along the internal elastic lamina of small arteries, and when neutrophils arrive, this layer disrupts. Elastase is the only known neutrophil enzyme that could be responsible. The probable role of elastase as a major proteolytic enzyme in pus is discussed below.

Collagenase is an enzyme that initiates the degradation of collagen from its normal triple helical configuration to the random coils found in gelatin.[17] It causes a scission of the molecule into two pieces, about 75 and 25% of the whole, respectively. Collagenase by itself does not degrade collagen much further, but the fragments are susceptible to several other proteases, including elastase, but apparently excluding cathepsin D. It would appear that collagenase is important in the dissolution of collagen that occurs in abscesses, and perhaps in the breakdown of other structures containing collagen, such as glomerular basement membrane.

Human neutrophils contain about 10 times as much neutral protease activity as do rabbit neutrophils. One group of proteases has elastase activity, the other resembles chymotrypsin. Interestingly, the chymotrypsin-like proteases appear to be identical with the bactericidal cationic proteins described by Spitznagel. The lethal effect on bacteria does not appear to be due to proteolysis, however, because the proteolytic activity is destroyed by mild heat, while the bactericidal action is not (Chapter 7, ref. 45).

8.3. Abscess Formation

A number of neutrophil proteolytic enzymes act on substrates in the surrounding plasma and liberate substances that either increase vascular permeability or summon more neutrophils into the site, or both. The substances include C3a and C5a, IgG fragments, and several different kinins. Because the arrival of neutrophils is autocatalytic, the fate of any lesion will be determined by a balance between the extracellular neutrophil proteases and the serum protease inhibitors, especially α_1-antitrypsin. Proteases will continue to be released as long as neutrophils die or as long as there is material to phagocytose, especially if it is spread out on a membrane. If too many neutrophils arrive in a lesion, the proteolytic activity will outweigh the serum inhibitors, and more or less extensive breakdown of tissue will ensue.

This "balance theory" of abscess formation was well known to early workers, and was summarized by Opie in a classic review.[18] In 1864, Eichwald showed that pus contained products of proteolysis, and by 1880, it had been shown that patients with various purulent collections such as empyemas had protein breakdown products in their urine. Müller extracted purulent sputum, or fresh pus, with glycerine, and demonstrated a protease that was active at neutral or slightly alkaline pH. Opie showed that this proteolytic activity was antagonized by serum. He did some experiments by injecting turpentine into the pleural cavity of dogs. Small doses excited a profuse exudative reaction and relatively few neutrophils; such fluids did not contain proteolytic activity. Larger doses attracted more cells, a point at which the serum proteins in the exudate could no longer antagonize the proteolytic activity of the cells was reached, and a sterile empyema resulted. In retrospect, he seems to have been investigating the elastase–α_1-antitrypsin system.

An abscess is a confession of failure: the consequence of inability to eradicate organisms by phagocytosis alone. It is perfectly clear that the necrosis of tissue is due almost entirely to the activity of the host's phagocytic cells, mostly neutrophils. In the first place, abscesses can be induced by injecting sterile irritants. In the second place, a series of workers, starting with Rich and McKee in 1937, have shown that in animals deprived of their neutrophils, there is little or no tendency to abscess formation when organisms are injected under the skin.[19] Rather, there develops an edematous, rapidly spreading infection that culminates in septicemia and the death of the animal. The same lack of localization is seen in infections of the skin in people with acute leukemia.

A general criticism of this type of experiment—a criticism that applies to almost all the data to be quoted in this chapter—is that it is not possible to distinguish between the consequences of lack of neutrophils and the consequences of lack of monocytes and macrophages. The macrophages in inflammatory sites are the descendants of blood monocytes that emigrate from blood vessels in the same way that neutrophils do. Monocytes also have a short half-life in the bloodstream (about 24 hr), and are constantly renewed by division of precursor cells in bone marrow. Procedures such as poisoning with benzene, nitrogen mustard, or cyclophosphamide, or X-irradiation, damage the precursors of both neutrophils and monocytes. When these procedures abrogate a response, it is therefore likely that neutrophils normally mediate it, since they are present in much larger numbers and may arrive in lesions quicker than do monocytes. However, one cannot be sure of this.

Abscesses probably arise only when there is some failure of the local defense mechanisms. The simplest is a huge inoculum of organisms. Experimentally, more than a million *S. aureus* must be injected into human skin to form a small pustule.[20] The required doses of several other bacteria are correspondingly large. Thus, under normal circumstances, when the skin and mucous membranes are intact, bacteria get into tissue only in small numbers, and are mopped up in detail before they have been able to multiply and without any noticeable local inflammation. Miles and his colleagues showed the existence of a crucial period in the first 4 hr of a bacterial infection, during which the fate of the lesion was decided.[21] Interference with the local inflammatory response by shock, or by epinephrine injections, could greatly increase the size of the lesion if they were used before 4 hr, but not after. Similarly, the inflammatory response could be inhibited by removal of the organisms with antibiotics, but only if they were used before 4 hr. It should be noted that at this time, there is hardly any local inflammation at the sites of bacterial infection; what seems to happen is that if the bacteria can multiply for a few hours, enough neutrophils will be attracted into the area to ensure the later development of an abscess. Since the bacteria are merely a trigger, they can then be removed without affecting the result.

When there is massive contamination of tissue through such lesions as a ruptured appendix or a compound fracture, local suppuration is inevitable. It can also occur with quite small inocula if some of the tissue is dead, or if there is foreign material in the wound.[20] Mixed bacterial populations are often more effective in overcoming the local defenses than are single species.[22] Infection of serous cavities, in which surface phagocytosis is impossible, may allow the buildup of a large local population. Finally, the local inflammatory response of the host may be suboptimal; causes of this condition range from neutropenia through defective chemotaxis to lack of opsonizing antibodies and complement components.

Once an abscess has developed, a new situation exists for both bacterium and host. On the one hand, the host has contained a large bacterial population in one place at the expense of some tissue necrosis. It is improbable that bacteria could get past the encircling ring of phagocytes into uninfected tissue. Pus is not a good growth medium for most organisms, and the bacterial population is high, so most of the bacteria are not growing. On the other hand, the bacteria are not dead, or die very slowly, and the highly proteolytic medium in which they are suspended would destroy antibody and complement opsonins even if the neutrophils could get at them. Furthermore, the osmotic pressure of pus is high, so abscesses tend to enlarge and to burrow along the line of least resistance. Frequently, this process leads to spontaneous evacuation through the skin, or into the bowel, with drainage of pus, collapse of the abscess walls together, and resolution of the lesion by scarring. However, a deep abscess such as an empyema or a subphrenic abscess may persist essentially indefinitely unless drained surgically. Eventually, bacteria may invade a blood vessel and cause septicemia, expansion of the abscess may compromise a vital organ, or the effects on the host's nutrition may wear down his resistance to the point where he can no longer keep the infection localized. There is no doubt that abscess formation is on the whole useful, but it is decidedly a second-best method of controlling infection.

8.4. The Arthus Reaction

The macroscopic features of the Arthus reaction were described in Chapter 5. This reaction was the classic type of Arthus phenomenon, in which the antigen is injected into the skin and the animal becomes actively sensitized. The essential feature is the combination of antigen with precipitating antibody in a skin site, and this combination can be arranged in two other ways. The passive Arthus reaction occurs when an animal is immediately sensitized by receiving an intravenous injection of precipitating antiserum from some other animal of the same or a different species. The reverse passive Arthus reaction occurs when the antibody is injected into the skin and the antigen is given intravenously.

Arthus reactions of any type are characterized by edema when they are mild and hemorrhage when they are severe. They remain soft, and lack the firm cellular infiltrate of delayed hypersensitive reactions. In very severe lesions, small blood vessels thrombose, and the center of the lesion becomes necrotic and ulcerates.

Histological examination, especially with the use of fluorescent antibody, shows that antigen–antibody complexes are deposited both in vessel walls and in the interstitium. Cochrane and Aiken showed that two principal places for deposition of complexes were the vascular basement membrane and the basement membrane of hair follicles.[10] Complexes were also deposited between the endothelial cells, with some protruding into the lumen. If colloidal carbon was injected about 1 hr after the reaction had started, it leaked out of the vessels, but was retained by the basement membrane. Fluorescent antibasement membrane antibody showed that the membrane was morphologically intact. After neutrophils had arrived in numbers, about 8 hr after injection, colloidal carbon leaked into the tissues, and fluorescent antibody showed disorganized basement membranes. These results were confirmed by electron microscopy. In animals deprived of neutrophils by nitrogen mustard or antineutrophil antiserum, the basement membranes remained intact. Further evidence that neutrophils are essential was provided by reconstituting nitrogen mustard–treated rabbits with neutrophils from a normal donor; they became susceptible to Arthus reactions. Also, as a rabbit's neutrophils returned spontaneously after nitrogen mustard treatment, he developed Arthus reactions at sites several days old. These sites contained antigen–antibody complexes, but had not reacted during the period of neutropenia.

The true Arthus reaction requires antigen and antibody to meet and precipitate in the vessel wall. If both antigen and antibody are put into the tissue, a much milder type of inflammation ensues, with less vessel necrosis. Antibodies that do not precipitate will not mediate the reaction, nor will those that do not fix complement. In fact, depletion of C3 by any of several techniques completely prevents development of the Arthus reaction, because neutrophils are not attracted into the sites.

8.5. Nephrotoxic Nephritis

A reaction identical in principle to the Arthus reaction is acute nephrotoxic nephritis, which occurs following the injection of antiglomerular basement membrane antibody, usually from another species. The antibody deposits linearly along the glomerular basement membranes, and this deposition alone produces mild proteinuria. However, the bound immunoglobulin itself is an antigen, and in due course, the host makes antiantibody, complexes form and fix complement, which attracts neutrophils, and severe nephritis results. Hawkins and Cochrane showed that fragments of glomerular basement membrane were found in nephritic urine.[23] In the first phase, these fragments were the same as those found in normal urine, but the quantity was increased. In the second phase, membrane fragments that had no counterpart in normal urine were found, and the presence of cathepsin E and probably D was also demonstrated. Since cathepsin E is found in neutrophils, but not in the kidney, it seemed likely that the neutrophils that could be seen lining the basement membrane were responsible for its degradation.

8.6. Serum Sickness

The acute form of serum sickness results from the intravenous injection of a large quantity of a foreign antigen.[24] A typical dose might be 250 mg bovine serum albumin per kg. For a week or so, the albumin is slowly catabolized, but then antibody secretion becomes significant, and immune complexes form in the circulation. Since there is a huge excess of antigen, these complexes are at first small, antigen-rich, and soluble. As more and more antibody is made, the complexes become larger, and when they reach a critical size, corresponding to a sedimentation constant of 19 S, they trigger histamine and serotonin release from circulating platelets and basophil leukocytes. This release increases vascular permeability, and the complexes leave the lumen and are trapped along the internal elastic lamina of small vessels. As more antibody is made, the complexes swing into equivalence or antibody excess, fix complement which attracts neutrophils, and vascular damage ensues, with disorganization of the internal elastic lamina as a prominent feature. The evidence that neutrophils are essential for vascular damage is similar to that for the Arthus reaction. There is a curious contrast between the arteritis and the nephritis of serum sickness.

Complexes lodge against glomerular basement membrane and fix complement in a manner apparently identical to that in the small vessels. However, the nephritis is mild, neutrophil infiltration is not prominent, and
depletion of neutrophils does not influence what nephritis there is.

8.7. The Shwartzman Reaction

This reaction is a very curious phenomenon that is still not satisfactorily explained. The generalized form (GSR) occurs when an animal, usually
a rabbit, is given two large intravenous doses of a bacterial endotoxin. The
spacing of these doses must be not less than 8 hr, nor more than 48 hr; the
optimum is about 20 hr. The reaction consists of generalized intravascular
coagulation, and its hallmark is renal cortical necrosis secondary to wide-
spread thrombosis of intrarenal arteries. The first dose of endotoxin
induces a qualitative change in the rabbit that alters the way it responds to
endotoxin. No single dose of endotoxin, however large, will induce the
GSR in a normal rabbit. There is also a localized Shwartzmann reaction
(LSR), in which the first injection of endotoxin is given subcutaneously,
and the second intravenously. The prepared skin site then develops hemorrhagic necrosis secondary to thrombosis of its vessels.

The GSR and LSR are prevented by treatment with heparin, unlike the
Arthus reaction. Thus, these reactions are due to intravascular thrombosis,
rather than to inflammatory changes in vessel walls. They are also prevented by depleting the animal of neutrophils. This prevention was originally demonstrated by Thomas, using nitrogen mustard,[25] and has been
confirmed by many workers since.

Endotoxin activates the blood-clotting system as well as the complement and kinin systems, so there is no difficulty understanding why it
should cause intravascular thrombosis. Normally, however, fibrinolysis is
also strongly activated, and there is little or no accumulation of thrombi in
vessels. The action of the first dose of endotoxin in promoting thrombosis
could therefore have one of three explanations: Endotoxin alters neutrophils and makes them procoagulant; endotoxin alters the blood-clotting
system, so that the blood is more easily clotted; or endotoxin impairs
fibrinolysis. There is some evidence for all these possibilities.

Horn and Collins showed that infusion of large numbers of normal
neutrophils into normal rabbits would allow them to develop the GSR in
response to a single injection of endotoxin.[26] The GSR could also be
produced in neutropenic rabbits in the same way. Infusion of neutrophil

granules sometimes led to severe clotting by itself, and it was easy to provoke the GSR by a single injection of endotoxin.

Niemetz showed that neutrophils exposed *in vivo* to two injections of endotoxin 16 hr apart had markedly increased procoagulant activity.[27] The neutrophils shortened the clotting time of normal plasma or hemophilic plasma; thus, they appeared to act via the extrinsic blood-clotting system. If these neutrophils were administered into an artery, renal cortical necrosis resulted.

Endotoxin injections cause massive clumping of neutrophils and deposition of the aggregates in pulmonary capillaries. Electron micrographs of pulmonary capillaries show that at 24 hr, many of the neutrophils are degenerate, and granular material leaks out into the capillary lumens.[28] The azurophil granules have been shown to contain highly charged anionic sulfated mucopeptides that markedly enhance blood-clotting. The first dose of endotoxin also induces the formation of soluble fibrin monomer complexes.[29] These complexes can be clotted by neutrophil granules, and this activity is antagonized by heparin.

A simple-minded view of the GSR would thus be that the first dose of endotoxin produces a feltwork of degenerated neutrophils in the pulmonary and probably other vascular beds. These neutrophils contain procoagulant substances in their granules. At 24 hr after the injection, the bone marrow has restored the initial leukopenia; indeed, there is a leukocytosis. In the plasma circulate partially clotted soluble complexes of fibrin monomer resulting from the first injection. The fibrinogen level is at least twice normal. Other effects on platelets and on fibrinolysis have been described and may be important. Into this highly unstable situation comes a second large dose of endotoxin. All the neutrophils are aggregated and dumped into capillary beds, where they degranulate or degenerate, or both, in either case exposing their granules to the increased supply of soluble fibrin monomer complexes also generated by the second injection. Platelets liberate factors that promote clotting, especially platelet factor 4, which is an antiheparin. The first injection of endotoxin has rendered fibrinolysis inefficient; hence, the platelet factors are not antagonized by fibrin degradation products as they usually are. The upshot of all this is massive intravascular clotting. The LSR presumably represents local clotting of soluble fibrin monomer complexes by neutrophils attracted to the skin site by the first injection of endotoxin. This scheme has the merit of explaining why both neutrophils and the clotting system are required for the reaction, but as stated, it is simple-minded.

8.8. Human Diseases Involving Neutrophils

There is much evidence that several spontaneous diseases of man involve the same mechanisms as those worked out in animals. In 1971, there was a diphtheria epidemic in San Antonio, and large numbers of children had to be treated with horse diphtheria antitoxin. Cases of serum sickness were to be expected, and a controlled trial of the value of antihistamines and antiserotonins was carried out in the hope that complexes could be prevented from lodging in vascular walls. The incidence of serum sickness in the treated group was one-fifth that in the controls.[30] A few cases of periarteritis nodosa, an inflammatory disease of arteries, have been attributed to complexes of hepatitis virus and antibody that were found in the lesions. Local Arthus reactions are seen at the sites of intramuscular injections of foreign sera. Generalized intravascular coagulation is seen in septicemic states, though renal cortical necrosis is rare except in pregnancy. This is of some interest, because pregnancy predisposes rabbits to the generalized Shwartzmann reaction.

Gout in humans appears to be caused by the liberation of lysosomal enzymes from neutrophils that have phagocytosed urate crystals. Crystals may be present in joint fluid at a time when there are no symptoms; it would seem likely that the serum protease inhibitors are dominant at these times. Gout is also much more common in men than in women. Weissmann and Rita showed that liposomes containing testosterone in their membranes were much more susceptible to urate lysis than were liposomes containing estradiol.[31] If it be assumed that lysosomes incorporate steroid hormones from their milieu into their membranes, a sex difference in sensitivity to urate might result.

Rheumatoid arthritis is peculiar in that it is a chronic disease characterized by a neutrophil exudate. The volume of exudate and the cell count may be unchanged for months or years. Hollingsworth labeled the neutrophils in the exudates of rheumatoid joints by injecting $DF^{32}P$ or $[^3H]DFP^{32}$. He found they had a half-life of only 4 hr, and calculated that a typical small effusion might turn over 10^9 neutrophils each day. Since the joint fluid contains antigen–antibody complexes and complement, there is obviously potential for phagocytosis, degranulation, and damage to joint tissue by neutrophil enzymes.[33] Many of the neutrophils in these joints are in fact degranulated, and enzyme release due to cell death must also occur, since cytoplasmic enzymes such as catalase and lactic dehydrogenase, as well as the usual lysosomal ones, can be found in the joint fluid. Neutral proteases that can degrade articular cartilage have been demonstrated in rheumatoid joint fluid, although it has not been shown for certain that they originate from neutrophils.

It is difficult to know how far neutrophils are involved in the pathogenesis of human glomerulonephritis. Animal data on the involvement of neutrophils in the pathogenesis of chronic glomerulonephritis are nonexistent, because of the difficulty of keeping rabbits neutropenic for any length of time. In human nephritides, immune complexes with or without bound complement can often be demonstrated in the glomeruli, and variable numbers of neutrophils are also found. Cochrane found that in nephrotoxic nephritis in animals, the neutrophil-mediated phase was associated with gross damage to the glomerular basement membrane. All proteins up to 1 million daltons leaked at comparable rates. On the other hand, selective proteinuria for small plasma proteins like albumin was found in the antibody-mediated stage. Proteinuria in human nephritis may be selective or nonselective, and in general, neutrophils are not prominent in glomeruli from kidneys demonstrating selective proteinuria. However, the converse is certainly not true; many grossly damaged kidneys show few or no neutrophils. Whether neutrophils were originally responsible for the damage is impossible to say.

8.9. Neutrophils and Tissue Repair

The alleged involvement of neutrophils in the repair of tissue has been completely disproved by Simpson and Ross.[34] They took ten guinea pigs and rendered them neutropenic by twice-daily injections of antineutrophil serum (ANS). The neutrophil counts of these pigs were all less than 300/mm³ throughout the experiment, and most of the counts in the first 5 days were less than 100/mm³. It is of some interest that three pigs died with frank peritonitis and two others were killed because they were obviously ill and were thought to be infected. Since the monocyte counts were normal, this result is evidence that the neutrophil in its own right is vital to antibacterial defense. One day after ANS had been started, six small sterile incisions were made in the skin of the back, and these incisions were removed for light and electron microscopy at 1, 2, 3, 5, 7, and 10 days. In neutropenic animals, no neutrophils were ever visible in the wounds, whereas they were plentiful in control animals. However, the number of monocytes, number and activity of macrophages, volume of fibrin, hyperplasia of fibroblasts, and synthesis of collagen were all entirely normal. The only differences noted were at 24 hr; the "space" in neutropenic wounds was less than normal, and the number of erythrocytes was greater than normal. Presumably, the "space" was occupied by edema fluid, and was diminished in neutropenic wounds because neutrophil enzymes were not available to activate kallikreinogens and mast cells and increase vascular permeability.

These studies appear to establish that neutrophils do not summon monocytes into wounds, nor play any part in their activation to macrophages. The fact that neutrophils do not influence fibroblast proliferation and collagen synthesis is confirmed by observations of Hill and Ward.[35] They induced mycardial infarctions in C3-depleted rats. No neutrophils entered the infarcts, but healing by fibrosis was normal.

8.10. Fever and Other Hormonally Mediated Responses to Infection

The body temperature in health fluctuates very little; it does rise to some extent with meals and with muscular activity, but if it is taken in the morning shortly after awakening, there are only small fluctuations from day to day. This constancy is maintained by a balance between the mechanisms that generate heat and those that dissipate it. Heat is constantly generated by cell metabolism in all tissues, and extra heat is generated whenever the tissue undertakes work. The work may be obvious, as in muscular exercise, or more subtle, as in the digestion of a meal. Heat is lost from the body mostly through the skin: by radiation, convection, and conduction, and through the latent heat required to evaporate sweat. We regulate our temperature primarily by our behavior: We do not go out in the tropical sun, or into snowstorms; we adjust our clothing to retain or lose heat; we have furnaces and air conditioning. Usually, we adjust so well that there is a rough balance between heat gained and heat lost, and body temperature is maintained constant by varying the amount of blood flow through the skin. If the small cutaneous vessels are dilated, the skin is warm and red, and heat is lost to the environment. If the small vessels are constricted, the skin is cold and pale, and heat is conserved. This adjustment of the rate of heat loss is adequate under all ordinary circumstances. Under conditions of heat stress, the emergency defense of sweating is called on; under cold stress, heat is generated by shivering.

This system is controlled by centers in the nervous system that are sensitive to blood temperature.[36] The principal centers are in the anterior hypothalamus and the preoptic area; they are bilaterally symmetrical. If this area is heated slightly, the animal vasodilates, sweats, and pants; if it is cooled, the animal shivers. Electrical stimulation of the anterior hypothalamus promotes shivering and vasoconstriction; removal of anterior hypothalamic nuclei produces an animal that cannot defend itself against heat stress. Recordings with microelectrodes have shown that the preoptic area contains neurons that are specifically sensitive to temperature, and that they increase their firing rate manyfold in response to a rise in temperature of 1°C. Thus, the anterior hypothalamic nuclei serve much the same function as a thermostat.

It has been known for more than a century that it is possible to produce fever by injecting pus into animals. Later, it became obvious that a wide variety of materials shared this property; some were of biological origin, such as milk or peptone, but some were inorganic, and even distilled water was noted to be pyrogenic on occasion. In 1910, Hort and Penfold investigated these fevers and showed that they could all be explained by contamination of the materials with bacteria. Freshly distilled water was not pyrogenic, but if bacteria were allowed to grow in it, they secreted a heat-stable substance that survived autoclaving and passed through filters that retained the bacteria that had made it. Siebert showed that only gram-negative bacteria secreted this substance, and we now know it to be endotoxin.

After this discovery, it was generally assumed that fever could be explained by endotoxin, but fever occurred in gram-positive infections, viral infections, and several conditions in which no infection of any type was demonstrable, such as rheumatoid arthritis, sarcoidosis, and Hodgkin's disease. Accordingly, many attempts were made to isolate an endogenous pyrogen from inflammatory lesions. Most of these pyrogens turned out to be contaminated with endotoxin.

In 1948, Beeson showed that saline extracts of rabbit neutrophils obtained from sterile peritoneal exudates contained a pyrogen that differed from endotoxin in that it was very heat-labile.[37] In 1953, Bennett and Beeson confirmed these findings, and showed that no other rabbit tissue contained pyrogens unless a neutrophil infiltrate was present.[38] Subsequently, it was shown that both human and rabbit neutrophils secreted pyrogen into the medium if they were incubated with endotoxin *in vitro*. By this technique, about 10 times more pyrogen could be obtained than was available by extracting the cells. Since then, pyrogens have been obtained from neutrophils of the cat, dog, sheep, goat, and monkey, and the list of stimuli that provoke their secretion *in vitro* includes phagocytosis of almost anything, myxoviruses, proteins to which a state of delayed hypersensitivity exists, DNA, and poly I:poly C.[39] It should be noted that many of these stimuli would be met by neutrophils as they go about their business in inflammatory sites. Furthermore, since both antigen–antibody complexes and proteins to which delayed hypersensitivity exists cause fever when injected intravenously, it is not difficult to understand why fever might occur in sterile inflammatory conditions such as rheumatoid arthritis.[39]

Fever does occur in diseases such as tuberculosis in which the infiltrates are composed mostly of lymphocytes and macrophages. It is also seen in agranulocytosis, in which there are few or no neutrophils in the blood or bone marrow. Atkins discovered that macrophages also had the capacity to secrete pyrogens in response to much the same stimuli as neutrophils.[40]

Neutrophil pyrogen is usually called *leukocyte pyrogen,* which was Beeson's original term. It appears to be a small protein, with a molecular weight of 14,000 daltons and a buoyant density in cesium chloride of 1.27. It is very labile, being destroyed by heat at 56°C for 30 min, and easily oxidized when exposed to air. It has been purified to apparent homogeneity by Murphy and his co-workers; their best preparations caused an average fever of 1°C in rabbits when 20 ng protein was given.[41] It is not known whether it contains any carbohydrate or lipid residues, and its amino acid sequence has not been determined.

Leukocyte pyrogen shows several biological differences from endotoxin, and procedures for totally inactivating endotoxin so that leukocyte pyrogen can be measured separately have been devised. Unfortunately, none of this evidence is absolutely conclusive. Stronger evidence that leukocyte pyrogen is not endotoxin was provided by Moore and his co-workers.[42] They were intrigued by the fact that neutrophils incubated *in vitro* put out very much larger quantities of pyrogen than could be obtained by extracting the cells. Three separate laboratories had showed that protein synthesis was essential for this pyrogen production, and that puromycin or cycloheximide would block it. This finding suggested that leukocyte pyrogen was actually synthesized *de novo* from amino acid precursors.

Moore therefore stimulated neutrophils *in vitro* in the presence of radiolabeled amino acids. The stimuli were endotoxin, phagocytosis of staphylococci, and tuberculin. The crude pyrogens were then purified to homogeneity. All the purified pyrogens were radioactive, and it could be shown by double-label experiments that the pyrogens made by neutrophils stimulated in different ways were identical. This result fits very well with the idea that fever is due to a specific molecule synthesized by neutrophils in response to suitable stimuli.

There is much physiological evidence that leukocyte and monocyte pyrogens are responsible for clinical and experimental fevers. Wood and his fellows worked with the rabbit, and showed that fever could be induced by the intravenous injection of endotoxin, gram-positive bacteria, and myxoviruses. In all these model fevers, and in the tuberculin and antigen–antibody-complex fevers investigated by others, pyrogen was found in the circulating blood.[39] This pyrogen behaved like leukocyte pyrogen rather than like endotoxin, and the quantity present was roughly proportional to the fever of the animal at the time the sample was drawn. In man, there are difficulties related to the amount of blood that can be withdrawn, but circulating pyrogen was demonstrated in severe febrile infections such as malaria and Rocky Mountain spotted fever. Endogenous pyrogens have also been found in inflammatory exudates in both rabbit[43] and man;[44] in the rabbit, it has been shown to get into the bloodstream via the lymph.

Since the anterior hypothalamus controls the body temperature, it would be logical to see whether leukocyte pyrogen acted on it. This determination was made very elegantly by Cooper in the rabbit[45] and by Jackson in the cat.[46] The results of the experiments were essentially similar. Intracerebral injections of leukocyte pyrogen caused fever only when given into the same tiny ($2 \times 3 \times 4$ mm) nuclei that were already known to be involved in temperature regulation. The quantity required to cause fever was only about $\frac{1}{100}$ that required by intravenous injection; furthermore, the time for the fever to begin to rise was reduced from 10 min to 2 min. Endotoxin caused fever only when it was injected in doses comparable with those required by intravenous injection. The time before fever began was 25 min or longer, and it was shown by histological sections that at this time a neutrophil infiltrate had developed at the injection site.

Wit and Wang showed that in animals given pyrogen, temperature-sensitive hypothalamic neurons lost their ability to increase their firing rate in response to a rise in blood temperature.[47] Furthermore, the well-known antipyretic aspirin restored the temperature sensitivity of these neurons to normal. This finding sounds very much as though the actions of leukocyte pyrogen on hypothalamic neurons are mediated by inducing prostaglandin synthesis. Several workers found that prostaglandins are pyrogenic when injected either into the hypothalamus or into the cerebrospinal fluid. Philipp-Dormston and Siegert therefore produced fever in rabbits by intravenous injections of endotoxin, Newcastle disease virus, or leukocyte pyrogen.[48]

By sampling the cerebrospinal fluid, they demonstrated increased levels of prostaglandins of the E and F series, which correlated with the observed fevers.

In summary, endogenous pyrogens are synthesized by phagocytic cells in response to stimuli commonly found in inflammatory sites. They pass into the bloodstream and change the behavior of hypothalamic neurons so as to induce fever. On present evidence, it would appear reasonable to conclude that all fevers are so caused except those due to lesions in the central nervous system. We have no idea whether endogenous pyrogens play any part in the normal regulation of body temperature.

There is a series of other responses to infection that are stereotyped and tend to occur in the same pattern regardless of the type of infection. Furthermore, they also commonly occur in noninfectious inflammatory conditions. During infection, iron and zinc are sequestered in the reticuloendothelial system, and if the infection is of any duration, the host may actually become anemic because iron is not available for hemogloblin synthesis. Also, there is an abrupt increase in the flow of amino acids into the liver; these amino acids are used to synthesize a group of proteins called the *acute phase reactants*. The best known of these reactants are the α_2-globulins, fibrinogen, ceruloplasmin, and the haptoglobins. The raised fibrinogen level is responsible for the elevated sedimentation rate; the elevated ceruloplasmin accounts for the elevation of serum copper reported in infection. A substantial part of the amino acid influx into the liver is used for gluconeogenesis; presumably, the glucose is used as fuel for the elevated metabolic rate characteristic of fever. The plasma amino acids are replenished by breakdown of protein in muscle and bone; this breakdown accounts for the muscle wasting and osteoporosis characteristic of severe infections.

There is evidence from studies by Pekarek[49] and Kampschmidt[50] that the sequestration of iron and zinc, and the metabolic changes in the liver, are mediated by a small protein secreted by phagocytic cells. The evidence is much less detailed than is that for leukocyte pyrogen, and much of it involves the use of rabbit material in rats. However, rat phagocytes secrete something that produces the same changes in rats, so the effects are real. Partial purification of these neutrophil supernates show that the proteins causing fever, iron and zinc sequestration, alteration in hepatic metabolism, and mobilization of neutrophils from bone marrow all are purified together, and as far as can be seen at the moment, appear to be caused by the same molecule.

One supposes that such an elaborate system of interconnected responses would not have evolved unless it were useful to an animal defending itself against infection. But it has so far been impossible to understand how any of these changes might be useful, and their disadvantages are manifest. In mammals, it is impossible to control the body temperature without provoking gross compensatory mechanisms that render interpretation of the results impossible. One recent experiment may have circumvented this difficulty. The lizard regulates its temperature entirely by behavorial means, and if it is placed in a constant-temperature enclosure, its body temperature equilibrates with that of its surroundings. Kluger and his colleagues took groups of lizards and maintained them in enclosures at 34, 36, 38, 40, and 42°C.[51] All lizards were infected with a constant dose of a bacterium pathogenic for lizards, *Aeromonas hydrophila,* and were observed for a week. Lizards maintained at 34°C were all dead by the fourth day; at 36 and 38°C, 20% survived; at 40°C, 65% survived; and at 42°C, nearly 80% survived. These are dramatic differences, and their importance is underlined by the fact that, left to itself, the infected lizard will regulate its temperature upward by 2°C or more. Thus, fever as a response to infection antedates the evolution of efficient temperature regulation, and it is likely to be an important defense mechanism, even if we are unable to say quite why.

References

References for the Introduction

1. Metchnikoff, E., *Lectures on the Comparative Pathology of Inflammation,* Translated by F. A. and E. H. Starling, London, Paul, Trench, Trübner and Co., 1893.
2. Metchnikoff, E., *Immunity in Infective Diseases,* Translated by F. G. Binnie, Cambridge, University Press, 1907.
3. von Behring, E., and Kitasato, S., Über das Zustandekommen der Diphtheria-Immunität und der Tetanus-Immunität bei Thieren, *Dtsch. Med. Wochenschr.* **16**:1113 (1890).
4. Pfeiffer, R., Untersuchungen über das Choleragift, *Z. Hyg. Infektionskr.* **11**:393 (1893).
5. Bordet, J., Les leucocytes et les propriétés actives du sérum chez les vaccinés, *Ann. Inst. Pasteur Paris* **9**:462 (1895).
6. Wright, A. E., and Windsor, F. N., On the bactericidal effect exerted by human blood on certain species of pathogenic microorganisms, *J. Hygiene* **2**(4) (1902).
7. Leishman, W. B., Note on a method of quantitatively estimating the phagocytic power of leukocytes of the blood, *Br. Med. J.* **1**:73 (1902).
8. Wright, A. E., and Douglas, S. R., An experimental investigation of the role of the blood fluids in connection with phagocytosis, *Proc. R. Soc. London Ser. B.* **72**:364 (1903).
9. Muir, R., and Martin, W. B. M., On the combining properties of opsonins of normal serum, *Br. Med. J.* **2**:1783 (1906).
10. Bulloch, W. B., and Western, G. T., The specificity of the opsonic substance in the blood serum, *Proc. R. Soc. London Ser. B* **77**:531 (1906).
11. Cowie, D. M., and Chapin, W. S., Experiments in favour of the amboceptor-complement structure of the opsonin of normal human serum for the *Staphylococcus albus, J. Med. Res.* **17**:57, 95 (1907).
12. Neufeld, F., and Rimpau, R., Über die Antikörper des Streptokokken- und Pneumokokken-Immunserums, *Dtsch. Med. Wochenschr.* **30** (part 2), 1458 (1904).

References for Chapter 1

1. Mahmoud, A. A. F., Warren, K. S., and Graham, R. C., Jr., Antieosinophil serum and the kinetics of eosinophilia in Schistosomiasis mansoni, *J. Exp. Med.* **142**:560 (1975).

2. Mahmoud, A. A. F., Warren, K. S., and Peters, P. A., A role for the eosinophils in acquired resistance to *Schistosoma mansoni* infection as determined by antieosinophil serum, *J. Exp. Med.* **142**:805 (1975).

References for Chapter 2

1. Cline, M. J., Isolation and characterization of RNA from human leukocytes, *J. Lab. Clin. Med.* **68**:33 (1966).
2. Cohn, Z. A., and Morse, S. I., Functional and metabolic properties of polymorphonuclear leukocytes. I. Observations on the requirements and consequences of particle ingestion, *J. Exp. Med.* **111**:667 (1960).
3. Kirschner, R. H., Getz, G. S., and Evans, A. E., Leukocyte mitochondria: Function and biogenesis, *Enzyme* **13**:56 (1972).
4. Stjernholm, R. L., and Manek, R. C., Carbohydrate metabolism in leukocytes. XIV. Regulation of pentose cycle activity and glycogen metabolism during phagocytosis, *J. Retic. End. Soc.* **8**:550 (1970).
5. Winkler, K., Heller-Schöch, G., and Neth, R., Protein synthesis in Human leukocytes. IV. Mutual inhibition of amino acid incorporation by amino acids in cell suspensions and cell-free systems, *Z. Physiol. Chem.* **353**:787 (1972).
6. Tryfiates, G. P., and Lazlo, J., Human leukemic polyribosomes, *Proc. Soc. Exp. Biol. Med.* **124**:1125 (1967).
7. Baggiolini, M., Hirsch, J. G., and de Duve, C., Further biochemical and morphological studies of granule fractions from rabbit heterophil leukocytes, *J. Cell Biol.* **45**:586 (1970).
8. Masson, P. L., Heremans, J. F., and Schonne, E., Lactoferrin, an iron-binding protein in neutrophilic leukocytes, *J. Exp. Med.* **130**:643 (1969).
9. Spitznagel, J. K., Dalldorf, F. G., Leffell, M. S., *et al.*, Characterization of azurophil and specific granules purified from human polymorphonuclear leukocytes, *Lab. Invest.* **30**:774 (1974).
10. Ramsey, W. S., Locomotion of human polymorphonuclear leukocytes, *Exp. Cell Res.* **72**:489 (1972).
11. Carter, S. B., Principles of cell motility: The direction of cell movement and cancer invasion, *Nature London* **208**:1183 (1965).
12. Senda, N., Shibata, N., Tatsumi, N., *et al.*, A contractile protein from leucocytes: Its extraction and some of its properties, *Biochim. Biophys. Acta* **181**:191 (1969).
13. Stossel, T. P., and Pollard, T. D., Myosin in polymorphonuclear leukocytes, *J. Biol. Chem.* **248**:8288 (1973).
14. Tatsumi, N., Shibata, N., Okamura, Y., *et al.*, Actin and myosin A from leukocytes, *Biochim. Biophys. Acta* **305**:433 (1973).
15. Ramsey, W. S., and Harris, A., Leukocyte locomotion and its inhibition by anti-mitotic drugs, *Exp. Cell Res.* **82**:262 (1973).
16. Peterson, S. C., and Noble, P. B., A two-dimensional random walk analysis of human granulocyte movement, *Biophys. J.* **12**:1048 (1972).
17. Ramsey, W. S., Analysis of individual leukocyte behaviour during chemotaxis, *Exp. Cell Res.* **70**:129 (1972).
18. Adler, J., Chemoreceptors in bacteria, *Science* **166**:1588 (1969).
19. Ramsey, W. S., Retraction fibers and leukocyte chemotaxis, *Exp. Cell Res.* **86**:184 (1974).
20. Zigmond, S., Mechanisms of sensing chemical gradients by polymorphonuclear leukocytes, *Nature London* **249**:450 (1974).

21. Tsung, P. K., Hermina, N., and Weissmann, G., cIMP and cAMP dependent protein kinase from human PMN leukocytes, *Biochem. Biophys. Res. Commun.* **49**:1657 (1972).

22. Bandmann, U., Rydgren, L., and Norber, B., The differences between random movement and chemotaxis; effects of antitubulins on neutrophilic granulocyte locomotion, *Exp. Cell Res.* **88**:63 (1974).

23. Allison, A. C., Mechanism of movement and maintenance of polarity in leucocytes, *Antibiot. Chemother. Washington D. C.* **19**:191 (1974).

24. Weissmann, G., Zurier, R. B., Spieler, P. J., *et al.*, Mechanisms of lysosomal enzyme release from leukocytes exposed to immune complexes and other particles, *J. Exp. Med.* **134**:149S (1971).

25. Ignarro, L. J., and George, W. J., Mediation of immunologic discharge of lysosomal enzymes from human neutrophils by guanosine 3', 5'-monophosphate, *J. Exp. Med.* **140**:225 (1974).

26. Elsbach, P., Increased synthesis of phospholipid during phagocytosis, *J. Clin. Invest.* **47**:2217 (1968).

27. Wurster, N., Elsbach, P., Simon, E. J., *et al.*, The effects of the morphine analogue levorphanol on leukocytes, *J. Clin. Invest.* **50**:1091 (1971).

28. Zucker-Franklin, D., Elsbach, P., and Simon, E. J., The effect of the morphine analog levorphanol on phagocytosing leukocytes—a morphologic study, *Lab. Invest.* **25**:415 (1971).

29. Smolen, J. E., and Shohet, S. B., Remodelling of granulocyte membrane fatty acids during phagocytosis, *J. Clin. Invest.* **53**:726 (1974).

30. Elsbach, P., Patriarca, P., Pettis, P., *et al.*, The appearance of lecithin ^{32}P, synthesized from lysolecithin ^{32}P, in phagosomes of polymorphonuclear leukocytes, *J. Clin. Invest.* **51**:1910 (1972).

31. Oliver, J. M., Ukena, T. E., and Berlin, R. D., Effects of phagocytosis and colchicine on the distribution of lectin-binding sites on cell surfaces, *Proc. Nat. Acad. Sci. U.S.A.* **71**:394 (1974).

References for Chapter 3

1. Sainte-Marie, G., and Sin, Y. M., Morphologic aspects and kinetics of the formation of neutrophils and eosinophils, in: Gordon, A. S. (ed.), *Regulation of Hematopoiesis,* Vol. 2, New York, Appleton–Century–Crofts, 1970, p. 1109.

2. Bainton, D. F., Ullyot, J. L., and Farquhar, M. G., The development of neutrophilic polymorphonuclear leukocytes in human bone marrow, *J. Exp. Med.* **134**:907 (1971).

3. Lichtman, M. A., and Weed, R. I., Alteration of the cell periphery during maturation: Relationship to cell function, *Blood* **39**:301 (1972).

4. Weiss, L., Transmural cellular passage in vascular sinuses of rat bone marrow, *Blood* **36**:189 (1970).

5. Killman, S.-A., Cronkite, E. P., Fleidner, T. M., *et al.*, Duration of some phases of erythrocytic and granulocytic proliferation computed from mitotic indices, *Blood* **24**:267 (1964).

6. Cronkite, E. P., Bond, V. P., Fleidner, T.M., *et al.*, The use of tritiated thymidine in the study of haemopoietic cell proliferation, in: *Haemopoiesis,* Ciba Foundation Symposium, London, 1960, p. 70.

7. Gilbert, C. W., The labelled mitoses curve and the estimation of the parameters of the cell cycle, *Cell Tissue Kinet.* **5**:53 (1972).

8. Monette, F. C., Lo Bue, J., Chan, P.-C., *et al.*, DNA synthesis time and related parameters in erythroid cell precursors of rats, *Scand. J. Haematol.* **5**:325 (1968).
9. Maloney, M. A., Patt, H. M., and Lund, J. E., Granulocyte dynamics and the question of ineffective granulopoiesis, *Cell Tissue Kinet.* **4**:201 (1971).
10. Constable, T. B., and Blackett, N. M., The cell population kinetics of neutrophilic cells, *Cell Tissue Kinet.* **5**:289 (1972).
11. Cartwright, G. E., Athens, J. W., and Wintrobe, M. M., The kinetics of granulopoiesis in normal man, *Blood* **24**:780 (1964).
12. Fleidner, T. M., Cronkite, E. P., and Robertson, J. S., Senescence and random loss of neutrophilic granulocytes, *Blood* **24**:402 (1964).
13. Perry, S., Weinstein, I. M., Craddock, C. G., *et al.*, The combined use of typhoid vaccine and ^{32}P labelling to assess myelopoiesis, *Blood* **12**:549 (1957).
14. Becker, A. M., McCulloch, E. A., and Till, J. E., Cytological demonstration of the clonal nature of spleen colonies derived from transplanted mouse marrow cells, *Nature London* **197**:452 (1963).
15. Trentin, J. J., Wolf, N., Chang, W., *et al.*, Antibody production by mice repopulated with limited numbers of lymphoid cell precursors, *J. Immunol.* **98**:1326 (1967).
16. Becker, A. J., McCulloch, E. A., Siminovitch, L., *et al.*, The effect of differing demands for blood cell production on DNA synthesis by hemopoietic colony forming cells of mice, *Blood* **26**:296 (1965).
17. Bradley, T. R., and Metcalf, D., The growth of mouse bone marrow cells *in vitro*, *Aust. J. Exp. Biol. Med. Sci.* **44**:287 (1966).
18. Metcalf, D., Transformation of granulocytes to macrophages in bone marrow colonies *in vitro*, *J. Cell. Physiol.* **77**:277 (1971).
19. Moore, M. A. S., Williams, N., and Metcalf, D., Purification and characterization of the *in vitro* colony-forming cell in monkey hemopoietic tissue, *J. Cell. Physiol.* **79**:283 (1972).
20. van Bekkum, D. W., van Noord, M. J., Meat, B., *et al.*, Attempts at identification of hemopoietic stem cells in the mouse, *Blood* **38**:547 (1971).

References for Chapter 4

1. Godwin, K. O., Fraser, F. J., and Ibbotson, R. N., Haematological observations on healthy (SPF) rats, *Br. J. Exp. Pathol.* **45**:514 (1964).
2. Fleidner, T. M., Fache, I., and Adolphi, C., Über die Umsatzkinetik der Leukocyten bei keimbreien Mäusen, *Schweiz. Med. Wochenschr.* **96**:1236 (1966).
3. Boggs, D. R., Cheverick, P. A., Marsh, J. C., *et al.*, Granulocytopoiesis in germ-free mice, *Proc. Soc. Exp. Biol. Med.* **125**:325 (1967).
4. Schulz, R. Z., Warren, M. F., and Drinker, C. K., The passage of virulent type III pneumococci from the respiratory tract of rabbits into the lymphatics and blood, *J. Exp. Med.* **68**:251 (1938).
5. Ambrus, C. M., and Ambrus, J. L., Regulation of the leukocyte level, *Ann. N.Y. Acad. Sci.* **77**:445 (1959).
6. Galbraith, P. R., Valberg, L. S., and Brown, M., Patterns of granulocyte kinetics in health, infection and in carcinomas, *Blood* **25**:683 (1965).
7. Gordon, A. S., Neri, R. O., Siegel, C. D., *et al.*, Evidence for a circulating leucocytosis-inducing factor (L.I.F.), *Acta Haematol.* **23**:323 (1960).
8. Craddock, C. G., Adams, W. S., Perry, S., *et al.*, The technique of leukophoresis and the response of myeloid tissue in normal and irradiated dogs, *J. Lab. Clin. Med.* **45**:881 (1955).

9. Boggs, D. R., Cartwright, G. E., and Wintrobe, M. M., Neutrophilia-inducing activity in plasma of dogs recovering from drug-induced myelotoxicity, *Am. J. Physiol.* **211**:51 (1966).
10. Bullough, W. S., and Laurence, E. B., The control of epidermal mitotic activity in the mouse, *Proc. R. Soc. London Ser. B.* **151**:517 (1960).
11. Rytomaa, T., and Kiviniemi, K., Control of granulocyte production. I. Chalone and anti chalone; two specific humoral regulators. II. Mode of action of chalone and anti chalone, *Cell Tissue Kinet.* **1**:329, 341 (1968).
12. Paukovits, W. R., Granulopoiesis-inhibiting factor: Demonstration and preliminary chemical and biological characterization of a specific polypeptide (chalone), *Nat. Cancer Inst. Monogr.* **38**:143 (1973).
13. Rytomaa, T., and Kiviniemi, K., Chloroma regression induced by the granulocytic chalone, *Nature London* **222**:995 (1969).
14. Metcalf, D., and Moore, M. A. S., Regulation of growth and differentiation in hemopoietic colonies growing in agar, in: *Haemopoietic Stem Cells,* Ciba Foundation Symposium 13 (new series), p. 157.
15. Morley, A., and Stohlman, F., Cyclophosphamide induced cyclical neutropenia, *N. Engl. J. Med.* **282**:643 (1970).
16. Morley, A., Howard, D., Bennett, B., *et al.,* Studies on the regulation of granulopoiesis. II. Relationship to other differentiation pathways, *Br. J. Haematol.* **19**:523 (1970).

References for Chapter 5

1. Zweifach, B. W., *Functional Behaviour of the Microcirculation,* Thomas, Springfield, Illinois, 1961.
2. Atherton, A., and Born, G. V. R., Relationship between the velocity of rolling granulocytes and that of the blood flow in venules, *J. Physiol.* **233**:157 (1973).
3. Intaglietta, M., Pawula, R. F., and Tompkins, W. R., Pressure measurements in the mammalian microvasculature, *Microvasc. Res.* **2**:212 (1970).
4. Luft, J. H., Capillary permeability—structural considerations, in: Zweifach, B. W., Grant, L., and McCluskey, R. T. (eds.), *The Inflammatory Response,* 2nd ed., Academic Press, New York, 1973, p. 47.
5. Majno, G., Shea, S. M., and Leventhal, M., Endothelial contraction induced by histamine-type mediators, *J. Cell Biol.* **42**:647 (1969).
6. Majno, G., and Palade, G. E., Studies on inflammation. I. The effect of histamine and serotonin on vascular permeability: An electron microscopic study. II. The site of action of histamine and serotonin along the vascular tree: A topographic study, *J. Biophys. Biochem. Cytol.* **11**:571, 607 (1961).
7. Wilhelm, D. L., and Mason, B., The role of endogenous permeability factors in mild thermal injury, *Br. J. Exp. Pathol.* **41**:487 (1960).
8. Marchesi, V. T., and Florey, H. W., Electron microscopic observations on the emigration of leukocytes, *Q. J. Exp. Physiol.* **45**:343 (1960).
9. Grant, L., and Epstein, F., apparently unpublished; quoted in: *The Inflammatory Process,* 2nd ed. (see ref. 4), Chap. 1, p. 34.
10. Williamson, J. R., and Grisham, J. W., Leukocytic emigration from inflamed capillaries, *Nature* **188**:1203 (1960).
11. Florey, H. W., Inflammation in: Florey, H. W. (ed.), *General Pathology,* Saunders, Philadelphia, 1970, Chap. 3, p. 103.

12. Spector, W. G., and Willoughby, D. A., The inflammatory response, *Bacteriol. Rev.* **27:**117 (1963).
13. Cochrane, C. G., and Wuepper, K. D., The first component of the kinin forming system in human and rabbit plasma. Its relationship to the Hageman factor, *J. Exp. Med.* **134:**986 (1971).
14. Spragg, J., and Austen, K. W., The preparation of human kininogen. II. Further characterization of purified human kininogen, *J. Immunol.* **107:**1512 (1971).
15. di Rosa, M., Giroud, J. P., and Willoughby, D. A., Studies of the mediators of the acute inflammatory response induced in rats in different sites by carrageenan and turpentine. *J. Pathol.* **104:**15 (1971).
16. Vane, J. R., Inhibition of prostaglandin synthesis as a mechanism of action for aspirin-like drugs, *Nature London New Biol.* **231:**232 (1971).
17. Hurley, J. V., *Acute Inflammation,* Williams and Wilkins, Baltimore, 1972, Chap. 5, p. 33.
18. Dukes, M., Chan, W. C., and Willoughby, D. A., The effect of various immunosuppressive agents on the vascular and cellular response to carrageenan in the rat, *J. Pathol.* **109:**151 (1973).
19. Kaley, G., and Wiener, R., Effect of prostaglandin E_1 on leukocyte migration, *Nature London New Biol.* **234:**114 (1971).
20. Allison, F., Smith, M. R., and Wood, W. B., The inflammatory reaction to thermal injury as observed in the rabbit ear chamber, *J. Exp. Med.* **102:**655 (1955).
21. Harris, H., Mobilization of defensive cells in inflammatory tissue, *Bacteriol. Rev.* **24:**3 (1960).
22. Ryan, G. B., and Hurley, J. V., The chemotaxis of polymorphonuclear leukocytes towards damaged tissue, *Br. J. Exp. Pathol.* **47:**530 (1966).
23. Boyden, S. V., The chemotactic effect of mixtures of antibody and antigen on polymorphonuclear leukocytes, *J. Exp. Med.* **115:**453 (1962).
24. Gallin, J. I., Clark, R. A., and Kimball, H. R., Granulocyte chemotaxis: An improved *in vitro* assay employing ^{51}Cr labelled granulocytes, *J. Immunol.* **110:**233 (1973).
25. Keller, H. V., Hess, M. W., and Cottier, H., The *in vitro* assessment of leukocyte chemotaxis, *Antibiot. and Chemother.* **19:**112 (1974).
26. Zigmond, S., and Hirsch, J. G., Leukocyte locomotion and chemotaxis, *J. Exp. Med.* **137:**387 (1973).
27. Keller, H. V., and Sorkin, E., On the chemotactic effect of bacteria, *Int. Arch. Allergy Appl. Immunol.* **31:**505 (1967).
28. Mayer, M. M., The complement system, *Sci. Am.* **229:**54 (1973).
29. Wardlaw, A. C., and Pillemer, L., The bactericidal activity of the properdin system, *J. Exp. Med.* **103:**553 (1956).
30. Ward, P. A., Cochrane, C. G., and Müller-Eberhard, H. J., The role of serum complement in chemotaxis of leukocytes *in vitro, J. Exp. Med.* **122:**327 (1965).
31. Shin, H. S., Snyderman, R., Friedman, E., *et al.,* Chemotactic and anaphylatoxic fragment cleaved from the fifth component of complement, *Science* **162:**361 (1968).
32. Clark, R. A., Frank, M. M., and Kimball, H. R., Generation of chemotactic factors in guinea pig serum via activation of the classical and alternate complement pathways, *Clin. Immunol. Immunopathol.* **1:**414 (1973).
33. Snyderman, R., Phillips, J. K., and Mergenhagen, S. E., Role of C5 in the accumulation of polymorphonuclear leukocytes in inflammatory exudates, *J. Exp. Med.* **134:**1131 (1971).
34. Hill, J. H., and Ward, P. A., The phlogistic role of C3 leukotactic fragments in myocardial infarcts of rats, *J. Exp. Med.* **133:**885 (1971).
35. Ward, P. A., and Zvaifler, N. J., Complement-derived leukotactic factors in inflammatory synovial fluids of humans, *J. Clin. Invest.* **50:**606 (1971).

36. Wilkinson, P. C., Recognition of protein structure in leukocyte chemotaxis, *Nature* **244**:512 (1973).

37. Kay, A. B., Pepper, D. S., and McKenzie, R., The identification of fibrinopeptide B as a chemotactic agent derived from human fibrinogen, *Br. J. Haematol.* **27**:669 (1974).

38. Kaplan, A. P., Kay, A. B., and Austen, K. F., The appearance of chemotactic activity for human neutrophils by the conversion of human prekallikrein to kallikrein, *J. Exp. Med.* **135**:81 (1972).

39. Yamamotu, S., Yoshinaga, M., and Hayashi, H., The natural mediator for PMN emigration in inflammation, *Immunology* **20**:803 (1971).

40. McCall, E., and Youlten, L. J. F., Prostaglandin E_1 synthesis by phagocytosing rabbit polymorphonuclear leukocytes, *J. Physiol.* **234**:98P (1973).

41. Becker, E. L., The relationship of the chemotactic behaviour of the complement-derived factors, C3a, C5a and C567, and a bacterial chemotactic factor to their ability to activate the proesterase 1 of rabbit polymorphonuclear leukocytes, *J. Exp. Med.* **135**:376 (1972).

42. Goetzl, E. J., Gigli, I., Wasserman, S., *et al.*, A neutrophil immobilizing factor derived from human leukocytes, *J. Immunol.* **111**:938 (1973).

43. Ward, P. A., and Schlegel, R. S., Impaired leukotactic responsiveness in a child with recurrent infections, *Lancet* **2**:344 (1969).

References for Chapter 6

1. Ponder, E., The physical factors involved in phagocytosis, *Protoplasma* **3**:611 (1928).

2. Neufeld, F., and Etinger-Tulczynska, R., Beitrag zur Wirkungsweise der phagozytoseerregenden Immunokörper, *Zentrabl. Bakteriol. Orig.* **114**:252 (1929).

3. Vakili, C., Ruiz-Oritz, F., and Burke, J. F., Chemical and osmolar changes of interstitial fluid in acute inflammatory states, *Surg. Forum* **21**:227 (1970).

4. Bennett, I. L., and Nicastri, A., Fever as a mechanism of resistance, *Bacteriol. Rev.* **24**:16 (1960).

5. Wood, W. B., Smith, M. R., and Watson, B., Studies on the mechanism of recovery in pneumococcal pneumonia. IV. The mechanism of phagocytosis in the absence of antibody, *J. Exp. Med* **84**:387 (1946).

6. Ward, H. K., and Enders, J. F., An analysis of the opsonic and tropic action of normal and immune sera based on experiments with the pneumococcus, *J. Exp. Med.* **57**:527 (1933).

7. Smith, M. R., and Wood, W. B., Heat labile opsonins to pneumococcus. I. Participation of complement, *J. Exp. Med.* **130**:1209 (1969).

8. Smith, M. R., Shin, H. S., and Wood, W. B., Natural immunity to bacterial infections: The relation of complement to heat labile opsonins, *Proc. Nat. Acad. Sci. U.S.A.* **63**:1151 (1969).

9. Winkelstein, J. A., and Shin, H. S., The role of immunoglobulin in the interaction of pneumococci and the properdin pathway, *J. Immunol.* **112**:1635 (1974).

10. Pondman, K. W., in discussion following: Boyden, S. V., North, R. J., and Faulkner, S. M., Complement and the activity of phagocytes, *Complement*, CIBA Society Symposium, London, 1965, p. 216.

11. Johnson, R. B., Klemperer, M. R., Alper, C. A., *et al.*, The enhancement of bacterial phagocytosis by serum: The rôle of complement components and two cofactors, *J. Exp. Med.* **129**:1275 (1969).

12. LoBuglio, A. F., Cotran, R. S., and Jandl, J. H., Red cells coated with immunoglobulin G: Binding and sphering by mononuclear cells in man, *Science* **158**:1582 (1967).

13. Lay, W. H., and Nussenzweig, V., Receptors for complement of leukocytes, *J. Exp. Med.* **128:**991 (1968).
14. van Oss, C. J., and Gillman, C. F., Phagocytosis as a surface phenomenon: Influence of C1423 on the contact angle and on the phagocytosis of sensitized encapsulated bacteria, *Immunol. Commun.* **2:**415 (1973).
15. Unkeless, J. C., and Eisen, H. N., Binding of monomeric immunoglobulins to Fc receptors of mouse macrophages, *J. Exp. Med.* **142:**1520 (1975).
16. Stossel, T. P., Field, R. J., Gitlin, S. D., *et al.,* The opsonic fragment of the third component of human complement, *J. Exp. Med.* **141:**1329 (1975).
17. Foley, M. J., Smith, M. R., and Wood, W. B., Studies on the pathogenicity of Group A streptococci. I. Its relation to surface phagocytosis, *J. Exp. Med.* **110:**606 (1959).
18. Wood, W. B., Smith, M. R., Perry, W. D., *et al.,* Studies on the cellular immunology of acute bacteremia. Intravascular leukocytic reaction and surface phagocytosis, *J. Exp. Med.* **94:**521 (1951).
19. Hinz, C. F., Properdin levels in infectious and non-infectious diseases, *Ann. N.Y. Acad. Sci.* **68:**288 (1956).
20. Fearson, D. T., Ruddy, S., Scher, P. H., *et al.,* Properdin pathway of complement in gram-negative bacteremia, *N. Engl. J. Med.* **292:**937 (1975).
21. Johnston, R. B., Newman, S. L., and Struth, A. G., An abnormality of the alternate pathway of complement activation in sickle cell disease, *N. Engl. J. Med.* **288:**803 (1973).
22. Alper, C. A., Abramson, N., Johnston, R. B., *et al.,* Increased susceptibility to infection associated with abnormalities of complement-mediated functions and of the third component of complement, *N. Engl. J. Med.* **282:**349 (1970).
23. Hill, W. C., and Robbins, J. B., Horse anti-pneumococcal immunoglobulins—specific mouse protective activity, *Proc. Soc. Exp. Biol. Med.* **123:**105 (1966).
24. Najjer, V. A., and Constantopoulos, A., A new phagocytosis-stimulating tetrapeptide hormone, tuftsin, and its role in disease, *J. Reticuloendothel. Soc.* **12:**197 (1972).
25. Young, L. S., and Armstrong, D., Human immunity to *Pseudomonas aeruginosa*. I: *In-vitro* interaction of bacteria, PMNs and serum factors. II: Relationship between heat-stable opsonins and type-specific lipopolysaccharides, *J. Infect. Dis.* **126:**257, 277 (1972).
26. Bloch, H., Studies on the virulence of tubercle bacilli. Isolation and biological properties of a constituent of virulent organisms, *J. Exp. Med.* **91:**197 (1950).

References for Chapter 7

1. Kanthack, A. A., and Hardy, W. B., The morphology and distribution of the wandering cells of mammalia, *J. Physiol.* **17:**111 (1894).
2. Hirsch, J. G., Phagocytin: A bactericidal substance from polymorphonuclear leukocytes: Studies on the bactericidal action of phagocytin, *J. Exp. Med.* **103:**589, 613 (1956).
3. Cohn, Z. A., and Hirsch, J. G., The isolation and properties of the specific cytoplasmic granules of rabbit polymorphonuclear leukocytes, *J. Exp. Med.* **112:**983 (1960).
4. Hirsch, J. G., and Cohn, Z. A., Degranulation of polymorphonuclear leukocytes following phagocytosis of microorganisms, *J. Exp. Med.* **112:**1005 (1960).
5. Hirsch, J. G., Cinemicrophotographic observation on granule lysis in polymorphonuclear leukocytes during phagocytosis, *J. Exp. Med.* **116:**827 (1962).
6. Zucker-Franklin, D., and Hirsch, J. G., Electron microscopic studies on the degranulation of rabbit peritoneal leukocytes during phagocytosis, *J. Exp. Med.* **120:**569 (1964).
7. Stossel, T. P., Pollard, T. D., Mason, R. J., *et al.,* Isolation and properties of phagocytic vesicles from polymorphonuclear leukocytes, *J. Clin. Invest.* **50:**1745 (1971).

8. Bainton, D. F., Sequential degranulation of the two types of polymorphonuclear leukocyte granules during phagocytosis of microorganisms, *J. Cell Biol.* **58**:249 (1973).
9. Estensen, R. D., White, J. G., and Holmes, B., Specific degranulation of human polymorphonuclear leukocytes, *Nature London* **248**:347 (1974).
10. Romeo, D., Cramer, R., and Rossi, F., Use of 1-anilino-8-naphthalene sulfonate to study structural transitions in cell membranes of PMN leukocytes, *Biochem. Biophys. Res. Commun.* **41**:582 (1970).
11. Nachman, R., Hirsch, J. G., and Baggiolini, M., Studies on isolated membranes of azurophil and specific granules from rabbit polymorphonuclear leukocytes, *J. Cell Biol.* **54**:133 (1972).
12. Lucy, J. A., Lipids and membranes, *FEBS Lett.* **40**:S105 (1974).
13. Lucy, J. A., The fusion of biological membranes, *Nature London* **227**:815 (1970).
14. Selvaraj, R. J., and Sbarra, A. J., Relationship of glycolytic and oxidative metabolism to particle entry and destruction in phagocytosing cells, *Nature London* **211**:1272 (1966).
15. Mandell, G. L., Bactericidal activity of aerobic and anaerobic polymorphonuclear neutrophils, *Infect. Immun.* **9**:337 (1974).
16. Klebanoff, S. J., and Luebke, R. G., The antilactobacillus system of saliva. Role of salivary peroxidase, *Proc. Soc. Exp. Biol. Med.* **118**:483 (1965).
17. Klebanoff, S. J , Myeloperoxidase–halide–hydrogen peroxide anti-bacterial system, *J. Bacteriol.* **95**:2131 (1968).
18. Klebanoff, S., and Hamon, C. B., Role of myeloperoxidase-mediated antimicrobial systems in intact leukocytes, *J. Reticuloendothel. Soc.* **12**:170 (1972).
19. Klebanoff, S. J., and White, L. R., Iodination defect in the leukocytes of a patient with chronic granulomatous disease of childhood, *N. Engl. J. Med.* **280**:460 (1969).
20. Rossi, F., Romeo, D., and Patriarca, P., Mechanism of phagocytosis-associated oxidative metabolism in polymorphonuclear leukocytes and macrophages, *J. Reticuloendothel. Soc.* **12**:127 (1972).
21. Root, R. K., Comparison of other defects of granulocyte oxidative killing mechanisms with chronic granulomatous disease, in: Bellanti, J. A., and Dayton, D. H. (eds.), *The Phagocytic Cell in Host Resistance,* Raven Press, New York, 1975, p. 201.
22. Hohn, D. C., and Lehrer, R. I., NADPH oxidase deficiency in X-linked chronic granulomatous disease, *J. Clin. Invest.* **55**:707 (1975).
23. Curnutte, J. T., Kipnes, R. S., and Babior, B. M., Defect in pyridine nucleotide dependent superoxide production by a particulate fraction from the granulocytes of patients with chronic granulomatous disease, *N. Engl. J. Med.* **293**:628 (1975).
24. Fridovich, I., Superoxide radical and superoxide dismutase, *Acc. Chem. Res.* **5**:321 (1972).
25. Curnutte, J. T., and Babior, B. M., The effect of bacteria and serum on superoxide production by granulocytes, *J. Clin. Invest.* **53**:1662 (1974).
26. Allen, R. C., Stjernholm, R. L., and Steele, R. H., Evidence for the generation of an electronic excitation state in human PMN leukocytes, and its participation in bactericidal activity, *Biochem. Biophys. Res. Commun.* **47**:679 (1972).
27. Webb, L. S., Keele, B. B., and Johnston, R. B., Inhibition of phagocytosis chemiluminescence by superoxide dismutase, *Infect. Immun.* **9**:1051 (1974).
28. Mason, R. J., Stossel, T. P., and Vaughan, M., Lipids of alveolar macrophages, polymorphonuclear leukocytes and their phagocytic vesicles, *J. Clin. Invest.* **51**:2399 (1972).
29. Sbarra, A. J., Paul, B. B., Jacobs, A. A., *et al.*, Metabolic activities of the phagocyte as related to antimicrobial action, *J. Reticuloendothel. Soc.* **12**:109 (1972).
30. Klebanoff, S. J.. Role of the superoxide anion in the myeloperoxidase-mediated antimicrobial system, *J. Biol. Chem.* **249**:3724 (1974).
31. Lehrer, R. I., and Cline, M. G., Leukocyte myeloperoxidase deficiency and disseminated

candidiasis: The role of myeloperoxidase in resistance to candida infection, *J. Clin. Invest.* **48:**1478 (1969).

32. Miller, T. E., Killing and lysis of gram-negative bacteria through the synergistic effect of hydrogen peroxide, ascorbic acid and lysozyme, *J. Bacteriol.* **98:**949 (1969).

33. Karnovsky, M. B., Biochemical aspects of the functions of polymorphonuclear and mononuclear leukocytes, in: Bellanti, J. A., and Dayton, D. H. (eds.), *The Phagocytic Cell in Host Resistance,* Raven Press, New York, 1975, p. 25.

34. Cline, M. J., and Lehrer, R. I., D-Amino acid oxidase in leukocytes: A possible D-amino acid linked antimicrobial system, *Proc. Nat. Acad. Sci. U.S.A.* **62:**756 (1969).

35. Johnston, R. B., Keele, B. B., Misra, H. P., *et al.,* Superoxide anion generation and phagocytic bactericidal activity, in: Bellanti, J. A., and Dayton, D. H. (eds.), *The Phagocytic Cell in Host Resistance,* Raven Press, New York, 1975, p. 61.

36. Brune, K. Laffell, M. S., and Spitznagel, J. K., Microbicidal activity of peroxidaseless chicken heterophile leukocytes, *Infect. Immun.* **5:**283 (1971).

37. Penniall, R., and Spitznagel, J. K., Chicken neutrophils: Oxidative metabolism in phagocytic cells devoid of myeloperoxidase, *Proc. Nat. Acad. Sci. U.S.A.* **72:**5012 (1975).

38. Jensen, M. S., and Bainton, D. F., Temporal changes in pH within the phagocytic vacuole of the polymorphonuclear neutrophilic leukocyte, *J. Cell Biol.* **56:**379 (1973).

39. Muschel, L. H., Carey, W. F., and Baron, L. S., Formation of bacterial protoplasts by serum components, *J. Immunol.* **82:**38 (1959).

40. Rowley, D., Endotoxins and bacterial virulence, *J. Infect. Dis.* **123:**317 (1971).

41. Brumfitt, W., and Glynn, A. A., Intracellular killing of *Micrococcus lysodeikticus* by macrophages and PMNs, *Br. J. Exp. Pathol.* **42:**408 (1961).

42. Griffith, E., Mechanism of action of specific antiserum of *Pasteurella septica*. Selective inhibition of net macromolecular synthesis and its reversal by iron compounds, *Eur. J. Biochem.* **23:**69 (1971).

43. Zeya, H. I., and Spitznagel, J. K., Arginine-rich proteins of polymorphonuclear leukocyte lysosomes, *J. Exp. Med.* **127:**927 (1968).

44. Odeberg, H., and Olsson, I., Antibacterial activity of cationic proteins from human granulocytes, *J. Clin. Invest.* **56:**1118 (1975).

45. DeWald, B., Rindler-Ludwig, R., Bretz, U., and Baggiolini, M., Subcellular localization and heterogeneity of neutral proteases in neutrophilic polymorphonuclear leukocytes, *J. Exp. Med.* **141:**709 (1975).

46. Mandell, G. C., Intraphagosomal pH of human polymorphonuclear neutrophils, *Proc. Soc. Exp. Biol. Med.* **134:**447 (1970).

47. Strauss, R. G., Anomaly of neutrophil morphology with impaired function, *N. Engl. J. Med.* **290:**478 (1974).

48. Spitznagel, J. K., Cooper, M. R., McCall, A. E., *et al.,* Selective deficiency of granules associated with lysozyme and lactoferrin in human polymorphs with reduced microbicidal capacity, *J. Clin. Invest.* **51** (abstract 305): 93a (1972).

References for Chapter 8

1. Cohn, Z. A., and Hirsch, J. G., The influence of phagocytosis on the intracellular distribution of granule-associated components of polymorphonuclear leukocytes, *J. Exp. Med.* **112:**1015 (1960).

2. Weissmann, G., Zurier, R. B., and Hoffstein, S., Leukocytic proteases and the immunologic release of lysosomal enzymes, *Am. J. Pathol.* **68:**529 (1972).

3. Henson, P. M., The immunologic release of constituents from neutrophil leukocytes. II.

Mechanisms of release during phagocytosis, and adherence to non phagocytoseable surfaces, *J. Immunol.* **107**:1547 (1971).

4. Spitznagel, J. K., Advances in the study of cytoplasmic granules of human neutrophilic polymorphonuclear leukocytes, in: Bellanti, J. A., and Dayton, D. H. (eds.), *The Phagocytic Cell in Host Resistance*, Raven Press, New York, 1975, p. 77.

5. Henson, P. M., The immunologic release of constituents from neutrophil leukocytes. I. The role of antibody and complement on non phagocytoseable surfaces or phagocytoseable particles, *J. Immunol.* **107**:1535 (1971).

6. Henson, P. M., Johnson, H. B., and Spiegelberg, H. L., The release of granule enzymes from human neutrophils stimulated by aggregated immunoglobulins of different classes and subclasses, *J. Immunol.* **109**:1182 (1972).

7. Goldstein, I., Hoffstein, S., Gallin, J., *et al.*, Mechanisms of lysosomal enzyme release from human leukocytes: Microtuble assembly and membrane fusion induced by a component of complement, *Proc. Nat. Acad. Sci. U.S.A.* **70**:2916 (1973).

8. Becker, E. L., Showell, H. J., Henson, P. M., *et al.*, The ability of chemotactic factors to induce lysosomal enzyme release. I. The characteristics of the release, the importance of surfaces and the relation of enzyme release to chemotactic responsiveness, *J. Immunol.* **112**:2047 (1974).

9. Shirahama, T., and Cohen, A. S., Ultrastructural evidence for leakage of lysosomal contents after phagocytosis of monosodium urate crystals, *Am. J. Pathol.* **76**:501 (1974).

10. Cochrane, C. G., and Aiken, B. S., Polymorphonuclear leukocytes in immunologic reactions. The destruction of vascular basement membrane *in vivo* and *in vitro*, *J. Exp. Med.* **124**:733 (1966).

11. Odeberg, H., Olofsson, T., and Olsson, I., Myeloperoxidase mediated extracellular iodination during phagocytosis in granulocytes, *Scand. J. Haematol.* **12**:155 (1974).

12. Clark, R. A., and Klebanoff, S. J., Neutrophil mediated tumor cell cytotoxity: Role of the peroxidase system, *J. Exp. Med.* **141**:1442 (1975).

13. DeWald, B., Rindler-Ludwig, R., Bretz, U., *et al.*, Subcellular localization and heterogeneity of neutral proteases in neutrophilic polymorphonuclear leukocytes, *J. Exp. Med.* **141**:709 (1975).

14. Ohlsson, K., and Olsson, I., The neutral proteases of human granulocytes: Isolation and partial characterization of granulocyte elastase, *Eur. J. Biochem.* **42**:819 (1974).

15. Janoff, A., Human granulocyte elastase: Further delineation of its role in connective tissue damage, *Am. J. Pathol.* **68**:579 (1972).

16. Janoff, A., Mediators of tissue damage in leukocyte lysosomes. X. Further Studies on human granulocyte elastase, *Lab. Invest.* **22**:228 (1970).

17. Ohlsson, K., and Olsson, Ir., Isolation and partial characterization of two granulocyte collagenases, *Eur. J. Biochem.* **36**:473 (1973).

18. Opie, E. L., Intracellular digestion. The enzymes and anti-enzymes concerned, *Physiol. Rev.* **2**:552 (1922).

19. Rich, A. R., and McKee, C. M., A study of the character and degree of protection afforded by the immune state independently of the leucocytes, *Bull. Johns Hopkins Hosp.* **54**:277 (1937).

20. Elek, S. D., and Conen, P. E., The virulence of *Staphylococcus pyogenes* for man. A study of the problems of wound infection, *Br. J. Exp. Pathol.* **38**:573 (1957).

21. Miles, A. A., Miles, E. M., and Burke, J., The value and duration of defence reactions of the skin to the primary lodgement of bacteria, *Br. J. Exp. Pathol.* **38**:79 (1957).

22. Altemeier, W. A., The pathogenicity of the bacteria of appendicitis peritonitis, *Ann. Surg.* **114**:158 (1941).

23. Hawkins, D., and Cochrane, C. G., Glomerular basement membrane damage in immunological glomerulonephritis, *Immunology* **14**:665 (1968).

24. Cochrane, C. G., and Koffler, S., Immune complex diseases in man and animals, *Adv. Immunol.* **16**:185 (1973).
25. Thomas, L., and Good, R. A., Studies on the generalized Shwartzman reaction. I. General observations concerning the phenomenon, *J. Exp. Med.* **96**:605, 624 (1952).
26. Horn, R. G., and Collins, R. D., Fragmentation of granulocytes in pulmonary capillaries during development of the generalized Shwartzman phenomenon, *Lab. Invest.* **18**:451 (1968).
27. Niemetz, J., and Fani, K., Role of leukocytes in blood coagulation and the generalized Shwartzman phenomenon, *Nature London New Biol.* **232**:247 (1971).
28. Horn, R. G., and Collins, R. D., Studies on the pathogenesis of the generalized Shwartzman reaction. The role of granulocytes, *Lab. Invest.* **19**:101 (1968).
29. Hansen, M. S., Bank, N. U., Barton, R. D., *et al.*, Enhancement of blood coagulation by soluble fibrin complexes, *J. Exp. Med.* **141**:944 (1975).
30. Kniker, W. T., Buerra, F. A., and Richards, S. E. M., Prevention of immune complex disease by antagonists of vasoactive amines, *Pediatr. Res.* **5**:381 (1971).
31. Weissman, G., and Rita, G. A., Molecular basis of gouty inflammation: Interaction of monosodium urate crystals with lysosomes and liposomes, *Nature London New Biol.* **240**:167 (1972).
32. Hollingsworth, J. W., Siegel, E. R., and Greasey, W. A., Granulocyte survival in synovial exudate of patients with rheumatoid arthritis and other inflammatory joint diseases, *Yale J. Biol. Med.* **39**:289 (1967).
33. Zvaifler, N. J., The immunopathology of joint inflammation in rheumatoid arthritis, *Adv. Immunol.* **16**:265 (1973).
34. Simpson, D. M., and Ross, R., The neutrophil leukocyte in wound repair. A study with antineutrophil serum, *J. Clin. Invest.* **51**:2009 (1972).
35. Hill, J. H., and Ward, P. A., The phlogistic role of C3 leukotactic fragments in myocardial infarcts of rats, *J. Exp. Med.* **133**:885 (1971).
36. Hardy, J. D., and Bard, P., Body temperature regulation, in: Mountcastle, V. B. (ed.), *Medical Physiology*, C. V. Mosby, St. Louis, 1974.
37. Beeson, P. B., Temperature-elevating effect of a substance obtained from polymorphonuclear leukocytes, *J. Clin. Invest.* **27**:524 (1948).
38. Bennett, I. L., and Beeson, P. B., The effect of injections of extracts and suspensions of uninfected rabbit tissues upon body temperature of normal rabbits, *J. Exp. Med.* **98**:477 (1953).
39. Wood, W. B., The pathogenesis of fever, in: Mudd, S. (ed.), *Infectious Agents and Host Reactions,* W. B. Saunders, Philadelphia, 1970, p. 146.
40. Atkins, E., Bodel, P., and Francis, L., Release of an endogenous pyrogen *in vitro* from rabbit mononuclear cells, *J. Exp. Med.* **126**:357 (1967).
41. Murphy, P. A., Chesney, P. J., and Wood, W. B., Further purification of rabbit leukocyte pyrogen, *J. Lab. Clin. Med.* **83**:210 (1974).
42. Moore, D. M., Murphy, P. A., Chesney, P. J., *et al.*, Synthesis of endogenous pyrogen by rabbit mononuclear cells, *J. Exp. Med.* **126**:357 (1967).
43. Bennett, I. L., The fever accompanying pneumococcal infection in the rabbit, *Bull. Johns Hopkins Hosp.* **98**:216 (1956).
44. Snell, E. S., Pyrogenic properties of human pathological fluids, *Clin. Sci.* **23**:141 (1962).
45. Cooper, K. E., Cranston, W. I., and Honour, A. J., Observation on the site and mode of action of pyrogens in the rabbit brain, *J. Physiol.* **191**:325 (1967).
46. Jackson, D. C., A hypothalamic region responsive to localized injection of pyrogens, *J. Neurophysiol.* **30**:586 (1967).
47. Wit, A., and Wang, S. C., Temperature-sensitive neurons in the preoptic/anterior hypothalamic region: Actions of pyrogen and acetyl salicylate, *Am. J. Physiol.* **215**:1160 (1968).

48. Philipp-Dormston, W. K., and Siegert, R., Prostaglandins of the E and F series in rabbit cerebrospinal fluid during fever induced by Newcastle virus, *E. coli* endotoxin, or endogenous pyrogen, *Med. Microbiol. Immunol.* **159:**279 (1974).
49. Pekarek, R. S., and Beisel, W. R., Characterization of the endogenous mediator(s) of serum zinc and iron depression during infection and other stresses, *Proc. Soc. Exp. Biol. Med.* **138:**728 (1971).
50. Kampschmidt, R. F., and Upchurch, H. F., Effect of leukocytic endogenous mediator on plasma fibrinogen and haptoglobin, *Proc. Soc. Exp. Biol. Med.* **146:**904 (1974).
51. Kluger, M. J., Ringler, D. H., and Anver, M. R., Fever and survival, *Science* **188:**166 (1975).

Index